Home Healing
with
Nature's Medicines

Home Healing
with
Nature's Medicines

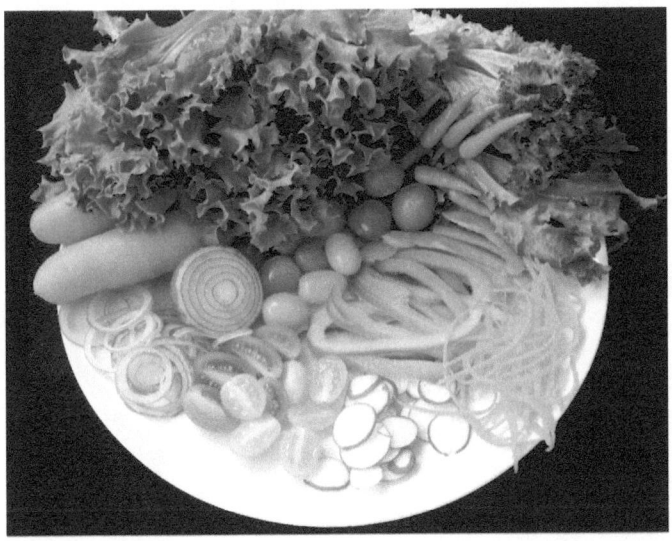

**A Hand Book of Home Remedies for Common Ailments,
Cures and benefits from fruits, vegetables, herbs and spices.
Exotic Recipes for healthy meals**

Shamim Ahmed

To order additional copies of this book, contact:
Xlibris LLC
1-888-795-4274
www.Xlibris.com
Orders@Xlibris.com
141553

Table of Contents

Dedication

I dedicate my humble work, this book, to my Creator, the Almighty God, the One Who gave me intellect, taught me, educated me and guided me in every step of my life. I reached where I am today with His help and with the support of my parents (May He give them best reward in the Hereafter).

Preface

Long before the advancement of science and the development of pharmaceutical products people relied on using natural things like leaves of trees, shrubs, and plants to cure the common ailments. They also used nuts, seeds, and roots of many plants, herbs and spices. Even some fruits are used to treat certain conditions. All these things are pure and natural with no harmful chemicals in them. There are no side effects to worry about. There is no harm in using these different things for common ailments before going to a physician. If they help you Praise to Almighty God! If these remedies will not help at least they will not harm you. Most of the things are found either in your kitchen or at any supermarket. Fruits are commonly available. Some herbs and spices you might have to look for at Chinese stores or Indian supermarkets. Not all fruits, vegetables, herbs and spices are covered in this book. There is lot of information for the seeker on internet, in libraries and book stores. But if someone wants a quick reference for very common ailments and the edibles that are good to maintain one's health then this book will serve the purpose.

Now a day there's actual scientific research that backs up some of these home treatments. Some of them ease tension, forestall headaches, and ease pain. Some of them work wonders on minor problems. Some of them are good to maintain good health, and give you immediate results but some of them should be used for a longer period of time to take care of the problem. Even more some of the herbs are approved by FDA as safe to use. Try to save your trip to the physician. Save your money and time. I am not giving any diet plan to anyone. It's all about keeping up with good health, and before any ailment or disease becomes chronic try these home remedies. They may be beneficial for your ailment. These are not a 100 percent sure treatment. But most of these remedies are tested by many people and they say they work. One of them might work for you.

This book is intended to be a quick reference book, more like a handbook that can be consulted easily. It's not like a heavy hard cover library edition that stays most of the time on the shelf.

You will also find some recipes of meals, with or without meat, salads and soups, at the end of this book. Keep up with Healthy Living.

Introduction

In medical profession the idea is that family doctors are our primary providers. Come to think of it, but mostly women consult their mothers or grandmother, even their friends and neighbors before calling a doctor for common ailments. They like to try those home remedies first.

Some natural plants and roots we cook as a source of our meals, and use some herbs and spices to make our foods aromatic and delicious. These things make our daily meals tasty and healthy. We need to live healthy. We should use what Nature has provided for us as medicines as well as to make our meals delicious.

However, in the last few decades there has been a resurgence of interest in natural medicine as an alternative to potentially dangerous pharmaceutical drugs. People are also trying not to use drugs that have dangerous side effects. Natural foods are source of Natural Medicine as well. If we avoid red meat all kinds of lentils, beans and some vegetables will provide the proteins our bodies need. If we need to take vitamins and minerals all kinds of nuts and seeds provide them. You can eat them and add them to your meals according to recipes. Vegetarian diets offer protection against many chronic diseases, especially constipation, cough, diarrhea, bug bites bad breath etc.

Use fresh and dry fruits, nuts and vegetables, herbs and spices. All are easily available in the supermarkets, Chinese or Indo-Pakistani stores. Eat health food to be healthy. I have selected only few items in each chapter. There is tremendous information about so many other things out there.

The key to a healthful vegetarian menu, if you want to avoid red meat, lies in eating a wide variety of greens and plant foods including whole grains, plenty of legumes, and generous amounts of fruits and vegetables. There are thousands of people in the world who are vegetarians and maintaining good health without eating any kind of meat. If you must, eat fish and lean meat. Avoid red meat occasionally. There are many of these fruits and vegetables, nuts and spices that help you get rid of many common ailments and discomforts for which we don't have to run to see the doctor immediately.

Ibn-Sina or Avicenna was a leading Arab physician (980-1037 AD). He wrote the "Canon of medicine". That was West's medical bible for 600 years. In Book Two he discussed the healing herbs. Nutmeg, senna, sandalwood, rhubarb, myrrh, cinnamon, cloves and rosewater were included in it. There is a remedy to many ailments that can be treated with different vegetables, fruits, nuts, herbs, and spices, and I have used many of them myself with good results. I have tried to compile those remedies from different sources along with what I was handed over by my older sister, aunt, and my mother.

Shamim Ahmed

Chapter 1

CURE FOR COMMON AILMENTS

In this chapter you will find remedies to those common ailments that so many people suffer from. Some remedies you may use while continuing your medicines prescribed by your doctor. Some try to use before you go to the doctor. If home remedy helps you save your time and money. Go to see a doctor if symptoms persist. Remember if you are a chronic patient of a disease these home remedies might not work. You would need more potent medicine.

1. Arthritis

Turmeric is a first rate anti-inflammatory herb. It is a commonly used in Indian sub-continent. Turmeric powder is used in preparation of different foods. Use about a ¼ spoon of it when making your meat dishes or certain vegetables. It has a strong yellow color that stains dishes and clothes that needs good cleaning.

The cartilage damage is associated with arthritis. It is partly caused by cell-damaging free radicals. Taking daily antioxidants are particularly effective at controlling free radicals. It's a good idea to eat foods (fruits, vegetables and nuts) that are rich in bioflavonoid.

- Taking recommended doses of vitamins A, C, and E daily will also help. Regular exercise and maintaining proper weight is also very important.
- According to the Arthritis Foundation, drinking tart cherry juice mixed with water three times a day may be beneficial for people with arthritis. This is due to its anti-inflammatory properties.
- Turmeric contains at least two chemicals, cur cumin and curcuminoids, that act to decrease inflammation linked to arthritis. Take ¼ of tea spoon at night with warm milk. It will

minimize the morning stiffness of joints. Half spoon of honey may be added to it. Drink mint and fennel seeds tea in the morning if it gives stomach discomfort. It will help.

- Half a teaspoon of cinnamon powder combined with one tablespoon of honey every morning before breakfast gives significant relief in arthritis pain after one week feel the difference and one could walk without pain within one month.
- Arthritis patients can benefit by taking one cup of hot water with two tablespoons of honey and one small teaspoon of cinnamon powder. When taken daily even chronic arthritis can be cured. Cinnamon tablets and capsules are also available at health stores and at pharmacies.
- Turmeric tablets and capsules are available at health stores and at pharmacies.
- Mix turmeric powder, fenugreek seeds powder and dry ginger powder of each of equal amount. Take one spoon with warm water every morning and every evening before bed time. In few weeks joint pain will be reduced considerably.

If you have persistent joint pain, then see an orthopedic physician.

2.   Asthma

A study has been shown that many children who eat Apples frequently had suffered less Asthma than those who have little or hardly any.

There are other anti-asthma foods. If used regularly, these foods will help reduce the effects of Asthma considerably: Avocados, broccoli sprouts, bananas, ginger, spinach, sunflower seeds, apple, rosemary, sweet potatoes, turmeric, mustard green, and kale.

Make ginger tea; drink it with a little honey added to it.

Make a salad with baby spinach leaves, broccoli sprouts, apple, avocado, and sprinkle it with some sunflower seeds. Use it regularly to reduce the effects of Asthma.

3.   Bad Breath

Bad breath is an upsetting situation and it is a common problem. When closely talking to people it is important to have fresh breath. People tend to avoid a person having bad breath. Bad Breath is caused due to some bacteria present in our mouth. These bacteria develop in the mouth during night when we are sleeping. There are many reasons of bad breath.

What causes bad breath?

- Lack of proper dental cleaning.
- Tooth decay
- Gum infection
- Bleeding gums
- Intestinal worms
- Constipation
- Leftover food in the mouth (Teeth not brushed after meals)

How you may get rid of the bad breath?

- Chew a clove after meals to get rid of bad breath.
- Chew cardamom seeds or sunflower seeds after meal. They are very effective in controlling bad breath.
- Chew fennel seeds after every meal to freshen up your breath.
- Gargle with warm water mixed with common salt. It removes bad breath and also clears the throat.
- Mix together baking soda and cinnamon powder. Scoop the mixture on to your toothbrush and brush away your bad breath after any meal.
- Use baking soda mixed with warm water to gargle that removes bad breath.
- Eating yogurt is also effective.
- After an hour of every meal brush your teeth or clean your mouth with lemon juice.
- Mint leaves help in removing bad breath. Chew a few mint leaves.
- Use commercial mouth wash to gargle.
- Chew cinnamon gum.
- Chew 'miswaak' to eliminate bad breath, improve sensitivity of taste-buds and to promote cleaner teeth. This was recommended centuries ago by Prophet Mohammad (peace be upon him). He also mentioned that using miswaak may eliminate as many as seventy mouth, gum and teeth diseases.

How to make your breath fresh?

Use *miswaak*. It is a teeth cleaning twig made from a twig of the *Salvadora persica* tree (known as *arak* in Arabic). It is a traditional alternative to the modern toothbrush. *Miswaak* is all natural, organic and green. It has a long and well-documented history of being reputed for its medicinal benefits. It also features prominently in Islamic jurisprudence of oral hygiene. It is used in different parts of Africa, Asia, especially the Middle East and South America. *Miswaak* sticks are used for oral hygiene, religious and social purposes and it does not need tooth paste.

Situations where *miswaak* is recommended to be used are: before religious practice, before entering one's house, before and after going on a journey, on Friday, before sleeping and after waking up, when experiencing hunger or thirst and before entering any good gathering.

In addition to strengthening the gums, preventing tooth decay and eliminating toothaches, *miswaak* is also said to halt further increase in decay that has already set in. Furthermore, it is said to create a fragrance in the mouth, eliminate bad breath, improve sensitivity of taste-buds and promote cleaner teeth. Besides there are 70 benefits of *miswaak* as suggested in Islamic Literature by Prophet Mohammad (peace be upon him) and many of these have been scientifically proven and the rest haven't been studied yet.

A few important benefits of *miswaak*

- Miswaak kills bacteria that cause gum disease.
- It helps effectively clean between teeth due to its parallel bristles.
- Miswaak cleans whole mouth including teeth, gums and tongue.
- It fights plaque effectively.
- It removes bad breath and odor from mouth.
- Miswaak also eliminates bad breath and creates a fragrance in the mouth.
- Increases salivation and hence inhibits dry mouth.
- Clears the voice.
- Removes the yellowing of the teeth.
- Whitens and make the teeth shine

Note: You can buy *miswaak* from Amazon.com.

Other ways to freshen your breath

- Eat less meat as it causes body odor and bad breath.
- Avoid eating raw garlic and onions.
- Keep up with dental hygiene.
- Have dental check up regularly.

- Use Listerine or any breath freshener. It is an anti-septic as well. You may buy breath fresheners without alcohol.
- Brush your teeth daily and if possible after every meal or you may use miswaak. You do not need to carry tooth paste, just the miswaak stick.
- Clean your tongue also. You may buy a tongue cleaner from any pharmacy.
- Drink lots of water.

4.   Bites and Stings of Insects

Bee sting remedies

- Pour a little honey on the affected site. It will cool the burning.
- Apply ice to cool the area.
- Mix baking soda and water to form a thick paste then slather it on the skin where the bee has stung.
- A drop of Lavender Essential Oils on the sting site will also cool it.
- People also use the bee balm and basil leaves.
- Slap a banana peel (the inside part) on an itch caused by a bug bite or poison ivy; this will bring down the inflammation and relieve the itch.
- Cut an onion in half and press the inside of it, the juicy part, on the sting.
- Crush a garlic clove to release its juices and press the crushed garlic against the sting.
- To get relief from pain of bee sting and wasp, apply lemon juice. Lemon can also act as mosquito repellent.

Spider bite remedies

The most effective remedy is the use of turmarind paste applied many a times a day on the bite. It will take a few days to heal the bite area. It's been tested with success.

5.   Blisters

- Listerine, used as breath freshener and an antiseptic, can also dry out blisters. Dab some on a cotton ball and apply it to your blister three times a day until it dries and the pain vanishes.
- Apply petroleum jelly on a blister for temporary pain relief.
- Use hydrogen peroxide, because it is antiseptic.

6. Body Odor

Close to people we have to be very careful of body odor. Some people have strong perspiration. Some perspire excessively. The underarm bacteria that causes body odor can be killed using home remedies. To keep you smelling fresh and sweet, instead of using expensive commercial deodorants, just use all-natural deodorants and have a sweet-smelling success.

- Take a shower every day using good deodorant soap.
- Witch hazel is very good for controlling body odor. Use it under your arms every morning after bath. It is also antiseptic.
- Tea tree oil is antimicrobial. Use it after morning bath to work all day long.
- Take 20 to 30 mg of zinc tablets daily. It is believed that zinc deficiency can cause people to sweat excessively. It is advisable to consult your doctor before taking zinc tablets.
- Apple cider vinegar changes the pH level to a higher level of acidity so that bacteria grow less readily. Use it on your salads.
- Replace fats and other cooking oils with olive oil or sunflower oil.
- Meats can cause body odor. Try to cut down their intake to minimal.

7. Cholesterol

Cholesterol is a kind of fat in your blood that is naturally formed in your body. It is normal, and essential to certain cell functions. But there are three kinds of fats in our body, LDL, HDL and Triglycerides we have to watch.

LDL is the cholesterol that is known as **Bad Cholesterol.** It is the major cholesterol carrier in our blood. But when too much LDL cholesterol circulates in our blood, it slowly builds up in the walls of the arteries. This buildup is called plaque. This LDL cholesterol can slow blood flow.

HDL cholesterol is known as **Good Cholesterol.** It is another type of fat called lipid found in the blood. According to the American Heart Association HDL cholesterol less than 40 mg/dL is low for men and less than 50 mg/dL is low for women. If your good cholesterol is low, your doctor may try to raise it, and LDL he will try to lower it.

Triglycerides are another type of fat in the blood. They are made in the liver and also come from foods that you eat. A high triglyceride level combined with low HDL or high LDL is associated with the buildup of fat in the blood. That's one reason why you should want your triglycerides to be lower.

How our home remedies and certain foods can help us lower our LDL?

It is said that some foods act like a burning machine for bad cholesterol or LDL. If we want to lower our LDL cholesterol then we should consider adding the following to our diet.

Nuts like almonds, pistachios and walnuts are a rich source of antioxidants and healthy fats (polyunsaturated fatty acids). Despite high calorie count moderate consumption of nuts reduces bad cholesterol. A light snack of almonds or walnuts in the morning is an easy home remedy to keep cholesterol levels in check. Just ½ teaspoon of cinnamon per day can lower LDL cholesterol. Ground flax seeds, brown rice, garlic, cinnamon, soybeans should all be in our daily use. Sunflower seeds, pistachios, pumpkin seeds, sesame seeds, pine nuts, flax seeds, and almonds are particularly high in plant sterols, which can help reduce LDL or bad cholesterol.

Fruits like grapes, strawberries and apples also come in the list of foods that lower cholesterol naturally. An orange every day is yet another way to bring cholesterol downward. A compound called pectin found in oranges and apples does not allow cholesterol to get absorbed into the bloodstream. Kiwifruit contains pectin, which has been shown to lower cholesterol. Plums have antioxidants that help prevent oxygen-based damage to fats. These include the fats that make up a substantial portion of our brain cells, the cholesterol in our bloodstream, and our cell membranes. A diet that includes a lot of cherries lowers all the overall risk factors for heart disease, including inflammation, body fat, and cholesterol.

Yogurt contains live cultures (good bacteria), that is excellent for binding bile acid (a byproduct of cholesterol). The good bacteria are instrumental in lowering cholesterol naturally.

Fish is high in omega 3 essential fatty acids and is considered to be one of the best cholesterol lowering foods. Add fish to your omega 3 essential fatty acids rich diet to raise good cholesterol and to reduce triglyceride levels. Just two servings of **salmon** every week provides adequate omega 3 essential fatty acids that ensure healthy cholesterol levels. Fish oil capsule may be used to bring down cholesterol.

Vegetables such as broccoli, lentils, kidney beans and peas are some of the soluble fiber foods that lower cholesterol levels. Oatmeal and oat bran are high in soluble fiber and help lowering cholesterol. The fiber in carrots helps to lower cholesterol levels. The magnesium in carrots also helps to regulate cholesterol.

Olive oil is equally important to keep cholesterol in the normal range. Olive oil contains some of powerful antioxidants and studies show that olive oil has the potential to lower cholesterol. It is better to change corn oil to olive oil for your cooking needs. Use it on salads. Use it in home-made salad dressings.

Orange juice, when consumed daily, is found to elevate good cholesterol as well as reduce LDL to HDL cholesterol ratio. But diabetic people have to be careful because of the contents of sugar in commercial juices.

Pomegranate juice reduces the size of plaque (deposits of cholesterol) in the arteries. It could repair the damage caused by arteriosclerosis (hardening of the arterial wall).

Cranberry and grape juices help in fighting high cholesterol and protect arteries from plaque building and prevent heart diseases.

Note: Drink these juices in moderation. It would be advisable to consult a nutritionist or alternative medicine physician before drinking too many different juices at a time. Even though these are nature's medicines and mostly do not have any side effects, using too many of them at a time is not advisable.

Drinking **tea** lowers low-density lipoprotein, the LDL. To help lower cholesterol and improve circulation, drink up to 4 cups of green and black teas a day.

If you do not want to have angioplasty or even bypass surgery, then try this natural therapy for opening veins and arteries of your heart:

- 1 cup lemon juice
- 1 cup ginger juice
- 1 cup garlic juice
- 1 cup apple cider vinegar

Directions

Mix all the juices and vinegar together and boil on low flame till it becomes 3 cups. Take it off and cool it down. Now mix 3 cups of natural honey and keep it in a clean bottle. Take one spoon of this juice daily before breakfast. Your blockage will disappear slowly. You have to take it consistently. At the same time, try not to eat any greasy or fried foods.

Eat more salads and fruits. Eat raw vegetables like carrots, cucumber, celery, radish etc. Walk daily or exercise at least for 20 minutes every day.

How you can increase your HDL?

Good cholesterol helps to build your body's cells. Increasing HDL cholesterol also can reduce your risk of heart disease. Most important thing is to change your life style.

- Reduce weight if you are over-weight.
- Try to quit smoking. Chose healthy fats like Omega-3 fatty acids, such as fatty fish, fish oil supplements, flaxseeds and flaxseed oil
- Eat whole grains, such as oatmeal, oat bran and whole-wheat bread and other products
- Use nuts, such as walnuts, almonds and brazil nuts for snack every day.

How we can reduce triglyceride level?

Triglycerides are fat the third kind of fat in the blood and are used to provide energy to the body. If you have extra triglycerides, they are stored in different places in case they are needed. If you get too much Fat collected in your belly you have high level of triglycerides. High triglyceride levels have been linked to a greater chance for heart disease.

Normal triglycerides means the level of them in blood should be less than 150 milligrams per deciliter (mg/dL).

Borderline high triglycerides = 150 to 199 mg/dL.

High triglycerides = 200 to 499 mg/dL.

Very high triglycerides = 500 mg/dL or higher. That means a dangerous level and high risk of heart disease.

To deal with high triglyceride levels is to eat a healthier diet and get more exercise. Moderate exercise on five or more days each week can help lower triglyceride levels.

- Losing weight can lower triglycerides. Belly fat is associated with higher levels. Try to reduce weight to a normal level, that should be according to your age and height
- Reducing saturated fat and trans fat in your diet can improve triglyceride levels and help manage cholesterol.
- Eat foods with low carbohydrates. It will also help lower triglyceride levels. Minimize the use of white rice, white bread, potatoes, pasta etc.
- Try not to drink alcohol, it can raise triglyceride levels. Some people with high triglycerides may need to cut out alcohol entirely.
- Eat more fish high in omega-3s. Fish like mackerel, lake trout, herring, sardines, albacore tuna, and salmon are high in omega-3s. If your triglycerides are very high your doctor may recommend a supplement or prescription omega-3s to lower them.
- Exercise regularly, even if it is a 20 minute walk in the back yard or on side walk.

8. Cold Sores

Cold sores or fever blisters are caused by the herpes simplex virus. They mainly occur on the skin adjacent to mouth, mostly on the lips. Sometimes they may occur on chin, nostrils, fingers or genitals. Cold sores are contagious. Canker sores are different. They are non-contagious mouth ulcer.

- Lemon balm can heal cold sores caused by the herpes simplex virus. This is not the herpes that is sexually transmitted. Once treated with lemon balm, not a single cold sore will have recurrence.

- Ice is a very good home remedy for cold sores. Rub ice on the infected skin for few minutes, repeat this every hour.
- Apply a tea bag for few minutes on the blisters; repeat this as often as you can. One can also consider pressing a warm tea bag on the blisters for as long as it stays warm.
- Witch Hazel on sores will give you some relief. Dip your moist index finger in powdered common salt and press the sore for 30 seconds using this index finger.
- Aloe Vera gel or oil is good way to heal the sores. People with weak immune system will take more time to recover and may face more severe consequences.
- Do not to attempt to disguise the cold sores by using makeup and other cosmetic products. Chemicals in them will simply cause further irritation to the skin and worsen the condition.
- According to many researchers licorice can actually help inhibit the development of cold sores. Sprinkle some licorice powder over the sores.
- Cold milk has a role in cold sore treatment. It can provide relief and even promote healing. Simply soak a cotton ball or swab in some cold milk and dab it or apply gently over the sore.
- Stress can trigger cold sores and one of the best ways to prevent cold sores is by sucking on zinc lozenges. These lozenges are very good for boosting the immune system and can therefore help in preventing cold sores.
- Use peppermint oil as it can penetrate the skin and it's powerful antiviral.
- A good home remedy for cold sores on the tongue is using Hydrogen Peroxide.
- Mix water with 2 ounces of hydrogen peroxide, one teaspoon of baking soda and five teaspoons of salt. Rinse the mouth 4-5 times a day with this solution. If you have sores on the tongue it would be very effective to get rid of cold sores.
- In case of severe cold sores, a cotton ball can be soaked for sometime in the plum juice and then used as a compress over the cold sores to relieve pain and inflammation.

9. Common Cold

- Use rosehip and ginger tea.
- Ginger and cinnamon tea with a few leaves of basil added at the end will also help.
- Use honey in place of sugar.

- In a cupful of boiling water pour a teaspoon of thyme and add a drop of peppermint oil. Sip slowly.
- Use lemon, oranges, and grapefruits to get as much vitamin C as you can. It will cure your common cold. Or just take vitamin C tablets 500 mg once a day.
- Basil seeds provide relief from influenza, fever and cold. Since it has antispasmodic effects, it can help treat whooping cough. In fact Tulsi (basil) is the main ingredient in many expectorants and cough syrups.

10. Constipation

Constipation is a common disturbance of the digestive tract. It is the chief cause of many diseases as it produces toxins which find their way into the bloodstream and are carried to all parts of the body.

Appendicitis, rheumatism, arthritis, high blood pressure, cataract, and cancer are only a few of the diseases in which chronic constipation is an important predisposing factor. From toddlers to the elderly any one can suffer from constipation. Chronic constipation can however be problematic and be indicative of other problems and of a faulty diet.

Causes of Constipation

Stress, anxiety or depression can contribute to constipation. Laxatives offer temporary relief. If suffering from constipation you need to make changes to your diet and your lifestyle for any lasting solution to the problem.

You can treat constipation with fruits:

- Try only one fruit at a time to see the results. If it does not work on your system then you may try another one or even two fruits every day.
- Patients suffering from chronic constipation should adopt an exclusive diet of this fruit or its juice for a few days. A **medium-sized pear** taken after dinner or with breakfast will also have the desired effect.
- **Guava**, wherever and whenever it is available since it is a seasonal and tropical fruit, is another effective remedy for constipation. It is eaten with seeds. It provides roughage and helps in the normal evacuation of the bowels. One or two ripe guavas taken every day will help the problem.

- **Grapes** have the properties of the cellulose, sugar, and organic acid. They make them a good laxative. Raisins are the dried grapes. When fresh grapes are not available, soak raisins in water in the night and eat them early in the morning, along with the water in which they have been soaked.
- **Oranges, papaya and figs** taken at bedtime and in the morning would be an excellent way of stimulating the bowels. Half a medium-sized papaya or 4-5 figs or 2 oranges will act as a very good laxative. It has been tried with good results.
- Both fresh and dry figs have a laxative effect. Four or five dry figs should be soaked overnight in a little water and eaten in the morning.
- We can eat fresh **plums** any time of the day. Prunes should be taken prunes in the morning and at bed time. Canned **prunes** in syrup are as good for the system as much as fresh and dried plums.
- Among the vegetables, spinach has been considered to be the most vital food for the entire digestive tract from time immemorial. Raw baby spinach contains the finest organic material for the cleansing, reconstruction, and regeneration of the intestinal tract. Use baby spinach in salads. Cooked spinach will be helpful for the problem.

Use these remedies as well:

- Warm cup of milk with one spoon of honey taken at bed time will help move the bowels in the morning.
- Squeeze half a lime or lemon in a glass of hot water, add half a teaspoon of salt, and drink it early in the morning. It is an effective remedy for moving your bowels.
- Drink the water, which has been kept overnight in a copper vessel, first thing in the morning.
- A teaspoon of linseed (alsee) oil swallowed with water before each meal provides both roughage and lubrication. Two teaspoonful of linseed oil may be taken at bed time instead.
- Sometimes a hot cup of tea early in the morning stimulates bowel movement. Many people like to have bed tea for this reason.
- Physical activity is good to regulate bowel movement.
- Drinking lot of water about 8 glasses daily as a routine is a good way of treating constipation.

Natural remedies and home treatments should be preferred, because repeating or frequent using laxatives can cause many other problems such as lazy colon syndrome. Body gets used to the laxatives and defection naturally becomes difficult.

11. Cough

Take a tea spoonful of honey with a pinch of ground black pepper on it at night before going to bed will subside cold. It may be repeated till cough is gone. It is tried with good result.

You may find cough medicine that is honey based at pharmacies by the name of Chestol.

Sauté freshly sliced garlic, without oil, till it is brown and crunchy, let it cool then grind it in to a powder. Put ¼ teaspoon on a teaspoon of honey and swallow it at bedtime. Cough will stop in 2 or 3 days' treatment.

Some of us have used Vicks VapoRub for years for everything from chapped lips to sore toes and many body parts in between. To stop night time coughing in a child (or adult), put Vicks VapoRub generously on the soles of feet, cover with socks, and the heavy, deep coughing will stop in about 5 minutes and stay stopped for many, many hours of relief. Works 100% of the time and is more effective in children, more than even very strong prescription cough medicines. It is extremely soothing and comforting and they will sleep soundly. Sometimes rubbing Vicks on a child's chest and behind the earlobes at night also help sleep better.

If you have grandchildren, pass this on. If you end up sick, try it yourself and you will be amazed at how it works.

Juice of raw and immature guava fruit or decoction of guava-leaves is very helpful in giving relief in cough and cold by helpful in giving relief in cough and cold by loosening cough, reducing mucus, disinfecting the respiratory tract, throat and lungs and inhibiting microbial activity due to its astringent properties.

Basil seeds provide relief from influenza, fever and cold. Since it has antispasmodic effects, it can help treat whooping cough. In fact, tulsi (basil) is the main ingredient in many expectorants and cough syrups.

12. Diabetes

Diabetes is very common these days. There are many factors that cause diabetes. It could be hereditary or it may be caused due to lot of stress. Diabetes A is more common among children and is also insulin dependent. Diabetes 2 is more common in adult.

In diabetes 2, your body either resists the effects of insulin or doesn't produce enough insulin to maintain a normal glucose level. Insulin is a hormone that regulates the movement of sugar into your cells. Diabetes must be treated. There's no cure for type 2 diabetes, but you can manage the condition by eating well, exercising and maintaining a healthy weight. If diet and exercise don't control your blood sugar, you may need diabetes medications or insulin therapy. Untreated diabetes can be life-threatening.

There are many home remedies to treat diabetes 2. First our intake of sweets, cakes, cookies, ice cream and any other sugary stuff should be controlled. Then you may try some home remedies. Keep checking your blood sugar levels. If home remedies are not helping then consult your doctor to give you prescription medicine.

- Bitter melon or bitter gourd is generally believed to be beneficial to diabetes. It is more popular in Asia to be used as a natural product for diabetes. Bitter melon has anti-viral and anti-neo-plastic activities. It shows moderate hypoglycemic effect of bitter melon juice, fruit or its dried powder. Thus, bitter melon may benefit certain people who are at risk of diabetes.
- Cinnamon may have a regulatory effect on blood sugar, making it especially beneficial for people with type 2 diabetes. Eating every few hours can help stabilize blood sugar, which is essential for diabetics. Cinnamon powder is readily available. Its tablets can be bought from any pharmacy. It is good for joint pain as well.
- Kiwifruit has Inositol, a sugar alcohol that naturally occurs in it. It may play a positive role in regulating diabetes. Inositol supplements may improve nerve conduction velocity in diabetic neuropathy.
- Okra is a commonly found vegetable. It is tested by some people to lower the blood sugar. Cut the top and the tail of okra, make two or three cuts on it and soak it overnight in half a cup of water. In the morning just drink the water. You may use the same okra for another day or you may throw away this one and use one other okra. If your blood sugar is too high then use two okras. You should continue taking your prescribed medicine. If you see considerable changes in your blood sugar level you may reduce your medicine to half. Keep monitoring your sugar levels. Consult doctor.

- The curry tree (Murraya koenigii) is a tropical to sub-tropical tree in the family of Rutaceae, which is native to India and Sri Lanka. Its leaves are used in many dishes in Indo-Pakistani vegetarian dishes. The leaves are generally called by the name "curry leaves". The leaves of Murraya koenigii are also used as an herb in Ayurvedic medicine. They are believed to possess anti-diabetic properties.
- India's traditional diabetes remedy from its native curry-leaf tree really does work, and could potentially be the making of a multi-billion dollar alternative drug, a landmark announced in British pharmaceutical conference. How to use it: Wash a curry leaves twig with about 20 leaves on it and boil it in 2 cups of water for 5 minutes. Let it cool and refrigerate it. Take 2 tbsp of that water every morning. Continue with your other medicine but keep checking your blood sugar. Within two weeks you should see the difference in blood sugar count going down.

Green juice for diabetics

A fellow juicer shared that he has been taking a tablet every night to control his blood sugar level. But, since he started juicing, he's been drinking this juice recipe every day. He's happy to say that after three weeks he could give up his tablet and his sugar level was stable.

Result may be different for different individuals.

Recipe

- ½ cucumber
- 1 green apple
- ½ bitter gourd
- 2 ribs of celery
- ½ green capsicum (bell pepper)

13. Depression

Depression can make you feel sad, helpless and uninterested in your favorite activities. There are many factors that may cause depression.

Physical, sexual and emotional abuse may cause depression. With many it may be mental illness. Sometimes hormonal changes may cause depression. Depression is more common in people whose biological family members also have this condition. Traumatic experiences in childhood may cause permanent changes in the brain that make a person more susceptible to depression.

If you suffer even from mild depression try one or some of fruits and see the results, and save yourself from medicines and their side effects.

Apple is one of the most valuable remedies for mental depression. The various chemical substances present in this fruit such as vitamin B, phosphorus, and potassium help the synthesis of glutamic acid, which controls the wear and tear of nerve cells. Take apple with honey and milk. They make an effective tonic that helps recharge the nerves and gives new energy and vitalize life.

The root of asparagus is highly nutritious and is used as an herbal medicine for mental disorders. It is a good tonic for the brain and nerves. One or two grams of the powder of the dry root of the plant can be taken once daily.

Have you heard the phrase "going bananas" because eating a banana facilitates the cross-talk among your brain cells and affects the mood? Preventing recurring minor depression banana a day therapy will help.

The use of cardamom is another thing that is valuable in depression. Boil water to prepare tea in the usual way and add some cardamom seeds in it. These seeds will add a very pleasant aroma to the tea, which can be used as a medicine in the treatment of depression.

An infusion of rose petals should be prepared by mixing half cup of rose petals in two cups of boiling water. Drink it occasionally, instead of the usual tea and coffee and get the benefit. If leave it to cool off place it in the refrigerator and drink it cool.

The cashew nut is another valuable remedy for general depression and nervous weakness. It is rich in vitamins of the B group, especially thiamine, and is therefore useful in stimulating the appetite and the nervous system. If you have weight problem avoid eating cashew nuts.

The herb lemon balm has been used successfully in the treatment of mental depression. It alleviates brain fatigue, lifts the heart from depression, and raises the spirits. A cold infusion of the balm taken freely is excellent for its calming influence on the nerves.

Peanuts are good sources of tryptophan, an essential amino acid which is important for the production of serotonin, one of the key brain chemicals involved in mood regulation. Surprisingly peanuts may have good affect in lowering the depression.

Diet has a profound effect on the mental health of a person. Nutritional therapy builds up brain chemicals, such as serotonin that affects the mood and are often lacking in depressed people. Eating foods that are rich in vitamin B, such as whole grains, green vegetables, eggs, and fish helps restore vitality and cheer in an individual.

The diet of a person suffering from depression should completely exclude tea, coffee, alcohol, chocolate, colas, all white flour products, sugar, food colorings, chemical additives, white rice, and strong condiments.

Regulate your diet habits to only three meals and no snacking in between. Eat fruits, nuts and seeds. Steamed vegetables, whole wheat bread, beans, lentils, milk, butter milk, salads etc should be the choices of your meals.

Be more active. Divert attention toward people and other things. Turn away from yourself. The pleasure of achieving something overcomes distress or misery.

Exercise is important in the treatment of depression. It not only keeps the body physically and mentally fit, but also provides recreation and mental relaxation. Exercise also tones up the body, provides a feeling of accomplishment, and reduces the sense of helplessness.

Yoga and meditation will help create a balance in the nervous system. This will enable the hormonal glands to return to a correct state of hormonal balance and will help overcome the feeling of depression.

If your depression still persists it's time to see a counselor and/or a physician.

14. Eyesight

Eyes are a very special part of our bodies. We have to protect our eyes, our vision the best way we can. We need not to put glasses on. We may even not wear contact lenses if we take care of our eyesight by eating the food that would protect our eyesight, far or near, getting bad, or getting any kind of diseases at our old age.

Lutein for the eyes

Lutein is a carotenoid vitamin, similar to vitamin A and beta-carotene. It is classified as a dietary antioxidant. Antioxidants help combat free radical damage to the cells. It is most often found in leafy green vegetables like kale and spinach. It is also prevalent in kiwi, squash, grapes, broccoli, corn and many more fruits and vegetables as well as egg yolks. Lutein is sometimes called the "eye vitamin" and actually functions as a color pigment in the human eye.

Eye health

Eating leafy green vegetables, kiwi, grapes, broccoli, corn, and eggs with yolks will actually provide the Lutein our eyes need. Intake of these things will protect the eyes from sun damage and oxidative stress. It may be essential in preventing eye diseases like cataracts, retinitis and macular degeneration.

Carrots are a great source of beta-carotene, which is converted to vitamin A in the body and is essential for eye health. It improves night vision and prevents age-related eye diseases like cataracts and macular degeneration.

Fourteen million American adults needlessly suffer from macular degeneration. Protecting our eyes is very important.

Dark circles around the eyes

Rose water has some natural properties to make the skin refreshed. That is why this is considered the perfect remedy to treat dark circles. Just take a cotton swab and dip it well into the rose water. It will kick off the dark circles.

Cucumber makes the skin refreshed every time we use it. Place slices of cucumber on both eyes encompassing the dark circle for about 15-20 minutes. They will absorb the heat from the skin and provide freshness and essential nourishment to the eyes.

Mint leaves, lemon juice, and tomato juice: This is very effective home remedy to cure dark circles. Moreover all the ingredients needed are easily available. Just take some crushed mint leaves and mix very little amount of lemon juice and tomato juice to make a tincture. Now with the help of a cotton swap apply this tincture on the dark circles and keep it for 10 minutes. Do it regularly to end the dark circle problem. Avoid eyes area. Take rose petals, the more the better, and put them into a cup of water. Boil then strain and put the water in a clean bottle. It will be very beneficial to remove the redness and weakness of the eyes. A weak tea is also good to wash your tired and red eyes.

Home remedy for eye health, and good eyesight

Take fennel seeds, almonds and sugar candy, in same weight, grind them to make coarse powder. Take a tea spoonful 2 or 3 times a day. Use it at least 6 months. Considerable improvement will be seen in the eye sight. In some cases people have gotten rid of their eye glasses.

Also use pistachios, carrot, apple, and beet root juices regularly. Spinach protects the eye from cataracts and age-related macular degeneration. Basil juice is good for night-blindness and sore eyes.

Check your and your children's eyes regularly, and make sure to give them the good diet from the very beginning to maintain their vision.

Proper diet will help enough not to wear prescription glasses from an early age if weak eyesight is not genetically inherited in the family.

15. Flu (Influenza)

Influenza (flu) is a viral infection. People often use the term "flu" to describe any kind of mild illness, such as a cold or a virus that has symptoms like the flu. But the real flu is different. Flu symptoms are usually worse than a cold and last longer. The flu causes a fever, body aches, a headache, a dry cough, and a sore or dry throat. A person will probably feels tired and less hungry than usual. The symptoms of flu usually are the worst for the first 3 or 4 days. But it can take 1 to 2 weeks to get completely better. Since it is viral there is really no medicine for it.

But there are many flu-fighting foods that will help get over flu fast.

Strawberries, cinnaman, turmeric, onions, raw garlic, raw honey, spinach, ginger, and cloves. Make teas with ginger, cinnaman or cloves or make it with ginger or red pepper. Use honey in place of sugar and drink sip by sip.

Use basil seed drink and basil leaves tea.

Eat the fruits and use other foods fresh or cooked.

Continue taking any medicine if doctor has prescribed it.

Basil seeds provide relief from influenza, fever and cold. Since it has antispasmodic effects, it can help treat whooping cough. In fact, tulsi (Basil) is the main ingredient in many expectorants and cough syrups.

Make a tea with red pepper or cayenne and take a teaspoon in a cup of hot water. Drink slowly before each meal and at bed time.

Boil heaping teaspoon of cumin seeds to each cup of water for 5 minutes. Strain when cool and add honey to taste.

Rub peppermint oil on the forehead, in front and back of the ears and on each side of the nose. Pour 3 to 4 drops in a bowl of boiling water and inhale through nose and mouth.

Remain in the house for a few days. Avoid meat. Adopt a vegetarian diet. Drink lots of warm drinks with flex seeds, mullein and slippery elm to excite a gentle sweat.

16. Headaches (Especially Tension Headaches)

Headache is one of the most common aches that most people suffer from. Headaches can happen to anyone irrespective of age and gender. Every time taking a painkiller is not a good idea. Try any of these home remedies for headache next time you get the headache before you take any pain medicine that has many side effects.

To prevent getting a headache you should do the following:

- Don't stay hungry for a long time. Hunger can cause headache.
- Eat green vegetables and fruits daily.
- Drink a glass of milk.
- Yoga relieves stress, maintains correct blood circulation and prevents headaches from occurring.
- Avoid eating junk and fried food as much as you can.
- A good night's sleep of seven to eight hours is a must to maintain balanced health.
- Eat a spoonful of sugar when you have a headache. The sweet sugar taste will give you instant relief from your headache.
- Avoid eating yogurt, cheese, and chocolate.
- Perform deep breathing exercises and half an hour walk daily.
- Do not suppress the natural urges, e.g. sneezing, passing stool and urine, hunger, thirst, sleep, breathing and yawning. They may trigger headache.

Home remedies for headaches

Following remedies are old-age remedies that have been practiced in Indo-Pakistan and Bangladesh.

- Make a paste with clove and salt and add it in the milk. Drink this milk. This drink will relieve the stress and the tension, which has caused the headache.
- Make a paste with water and cinnamon powder and apply it on the head and temples.
- Applying sandalwood paste on the forehead will also give relief from headache. This remedy should be tried in case you got a headache in summer due to the heat.
- Massage your head with coconut oil. This will help the blood circulation in the head thus give instant relief from headache.

- Massage your forehead with almond oil to get instant relief from the headaches.
- Massage olive oil on the palms of your hands. Surprisingly you will feel the headache is relieved.
- Drinking a cup of tea is also a very old method of curing headaches. Add ginger, cumin and coriander seeds while making the tea.
- Massage your head with eucalyptus oil.
- Every morning eat an apple with a pinch of salt added to it. Drink either water or milk with it. Do this regime for about ten days. This remedy is good for those who get headaches too often.
- Dab cotton ball in lemon juice and apply it on your forehead and temples.
- Drink herbal tea.
- If you get a headache due to cold, make a drink with sugar, cinnamon and coriander and drink it.
- Place your finger between your eyebrows, (this is a pressure point) press it and release, repeat three times. Place your both index fingers on each side of your temple, (another pressure point); press your fingers on your temple and release. Do it three times.
- A very funny and silly use of banana peel is to put the inside of banana peel on your forehead and on the back of your neck. Surprisingly it will soothe the pain.
- Get some coca cola or Pepsi and put salted peanuts in it and drink it as you normally would. Sometimes acidity causes headaches. In a glass of water squeeze ½ lemon and drink it. It is one of the best remedies for headaches. It also cures the acidity.
- Put Vicks VapoRub on temples; press the bridge above the nose with thumbs. For sinus headache put a spoon of Vick VapoRub in boiling water in a big bowl. Cover your head and the bowl with a towel and inhale the steam. Sinuses will open up and headache will be relieved.
- Buy Valerian root. It's actually a great pain medication and it's completely safe. Sometimes essential oils like peppermint oil, eucalyptus oil, tea tree oil, and lavender oil may be used to treat headaches.
- Drink as much water as possible.
- Apply olive oil to the hairline when have a headache. Press between the web of the thumb and index finger to relieve

headache. Take both hands and rub forehead, up to temples, with pressure in circles with your palms, then use finger tips. Go counter clockwise and clockwise and then opposite for about 5 minutes. It's a massaging technique, and will relieve headache.

If still headache persists then take any pain relieving medicine that suits you or your doctor has recommended it. Consulting your doctor for persistent and frequently occurring headaches is advisable. Severe headaches should not be neglected.

17. Heart Burn or Stomach Burn

The feeling of heart burn or stomach burn is when either you have eaten very spicy and oily food or you have indigestion.

- Drink ginger tea. Slice about a one inch piece of ginger; boil it in one and half cup of water. When water is about one cup left add a tea bag. Turn off the stove. Let the tea brew for couple of minutes. Add honey, sugar or lemon for taste and drink.
- Drink light green tea.
- Drink cold milk.
- Drink mint and fennel seed tea. Boil a twig of mint and half spoon of fennel seeds in one cup of water. Take it off the stove. Strain it in a mug. Add a tea bag. Let it brew for few minutes. Add lemon or honey for taste. You may add salt in place of sugar if you like the taste. Take small sips.
- Take 2 tablets of "Hajmola". You may buy it from any Indian sub-continental stores. It works!
- Some people heal heartburn with apple cider vinegar added to a glass of water taken before every meal. It is very effective digestive remedy.
- Make tea with fresh mint leaves and cardamom and a tea bag. Drink with or without sugar or honey.
- Boil a spoonful of fennel seeds in cup of water. Let it cool and drink warm. Add some salt and pepper to your taste.

18. Heart Disease and High Blood Pressure

I am not a doctor or any kind of medical professional. But I have many doctors and pharmacists in the family. I constantly talk and have discussions with them about heart disease and hypertension because these two ailments run in my family. I am a high blood pressure patient and constantly try to control it natural ways more than completely depending on medicines prescribed by doctors.

Elevated blood pressure is a major risk factor for heart attack and or stroke. Smoking and high cholesterol also contribute to possible heart attack. Periodically you must watch your blood pressure. Hypertension is defined as a blood pressure of 140/90. The top number represents systolic pressure. It is arterial pressure when the heart contracts. The second one is diastolic pressure. It is the pressure between heart beats.

If you are suffering from hypertension make no mistake of measuring pressure by the numbers. Everyone's blood pressure differs. Unreliable BP instrument should not be used.

Drinking alcoholic beverages may raise the pressure considerably. Some doctors advice their patients to drink only wine and in moderation. I would suggest avoid drinking any alcoholic beverage.

Not all patients have to cut down salt completely but it is better to minimize the intake of salt.

Exercise is very important. Regular exercise will reduce the blood pressure and the risk of heart attack.

Eat potassium-rich foods like bananas, oranges, squash, and sunflowers seeds.

Following fruits are good and very helpful in preventing heart disease and hypertension:

Papayas are a good source of 3 powerful antioxidants—vitamins C, E, and A—that prevent the oxidation of cholesterol and may prevent atherosclerosis and heart disease. They're one of the best sources of digestive enzymes that break down protein and may help reduce inflammation.

Kiwis contain twice the amount of vitamin C as oranges. Kiwis are a good source of fiber, which can help lower cholesterol and regulate blood sugar. They may also lower your risk for blood clots and reduce fats in your blood.

Spinach has shown to effectively lower blood pressure.

Clementines are rich in vitamin C that helps support the immune system. They're also a good source of calcium, a necessity for bone health, and potassium, which can help lower blood pressure.

Guava fruit being very rich in fiber and hypoglycemic in nature, helps reduce blood pressure. It is a tropical and seasonal fruit. If it is available eat one or two medium size guavas every day.

Remedies

Soak the rose flower petals in the water overnight and keep it in the refrigerator. Drink that water in the morning and after any strenuous activity.

These three different tastes make a great-tasting juice combo. This is nature's gift to help lower high blood pressure:

- 2 pears
- 2 ribs of celery
- 2 sour limes
- ice-cubes (optional)

Directions

Blend them in high speed blender and the drink is ready for you.

Prayer is a form of meditation that helps to slow down breathing and brain activity and reduces high blood pressure. Whenever you have a few minutes and a quiet corner pray or sit quietly with your eyes closed like you are in meditation.

Heart health and Lutein

Lutein is a carotenoid vitamin, similar to vitamin A and beta-carotene. It is classified as a dietary antioxidant. Antioxidants help combat free radical damage to the cells. It is most often found in leafy green vegetables like kale and spinach. It is also prevalent in kiwi, squash, grapes, broccoli, corn, and many more fruits and vegetables as well as egg yolks. A major human study of atherosclerosis showed that Lutein and other carotenoids may help prevent heart attack and stroke. Lutein can help prevent oxidative stress to cholesterol and the cardiovascular system. It may prevent thickening of carotid arteries. It may prevent clogging and thickness of arteries.

All the vegetables and fruits that Lutein in them make them part of your daily diet.

19. Kidney Stones

Kidney stones may form when the normal balance of water, salts, minerals, and other substances found in urine changes. How this balance changes determines the type of kidney stone you have. Most kidney stones are calcium type. They form when the calcium levels in your urine change.

In case of kidney stones, one teaspoon each of basil juice and honey should be taken daily till the stone are expelled from the urinary tract. Basil has a strengthening effect on the kidneys.

The seeds of both sour and sweet pomegranates are useful medicine for kidney stones. A tablespoon of the seeds, ground into a fine paste, can be given along with a cup of horse gram (kulthi) soup to dissolve gravel in kidneys. Two tablespoons of horse gram should be used for preparing the cup of soup. Pomegranate seed powder can be bought from Indian stores.

Celery prevents stone formation in kidneys and gallbladder.

Apple cider is very valuable in treating kidney stones.

Use of grapes is also an excellent cure for kidney stones.

Watermelon is also rich in potassium salts. It is one of the safest and best diuretics which can be used with beneficial result in kidney stones.

Drinking lot of water is very necessary.

Alcoholic beverages, condiments and pickles; certain vegetables like cucumber, radish, tomato, spinach, rhubarb; those with a strong aroma such as asparagus, onion, beans, cabbage, and cauliflower; meat and gravies; and carbonated waters should be avoided.

Kidney beans, also known as dried French beans or Rajmah, are regarded as a very effective home remedy for kidney problems, including kidney stones.

To prepare the medicine remove the beans from inside the pods, then slice the pods and put about sixty grams in four liter of hot water, boil them slowly for six hours. This liquid should be strained through fine muslin and then allowed to cool for about eight hours. Thereafter the fluid should be poured through another piece of muslin without stirring, till it is thoroughly distilled.

A glass of this decoction should be given to the patient every two hours throughout the day for one day. It may be taken several times a week. This decoction would work only when it is freshly made. Because once the beans were boiled their therapeutic effect would disappear after one day.

Cranberry juice is best known for its ability to protect against urinary tract infections. Cranberries have antioxidant and are anti-inflammatory.

The foods that may be irritant to the kidneys should be avoided: whole wheat flour, chickpea, peas, soy bean, beet, spinach, cauliflower, turnips, carrots, almonds, and coconuts.

Low-protein diet is better.

With the advice of a doctor a daily therapeutic dose of 100 to 150 mg of vitamin B6, preferably, combined with other B complex vitamins, should be continued for several months for getting a permanent cure.

20. Menstrual Pain

Many women suffer from menstrual pain. Some say it goes away after marriage and some say after child birth. But surly some women do not suffer from menstrual pain all their lives.

Anyway there are certain tips to help ease this menstrual pain. Avoid medicine if you can. Even most popular pain killers have side effects.

- Exercise and taking hot steamy bath are helpful in relieving pain. Use essential oils with it.
- Wear loose clothing. Enough space will make you feel relaxed.
- Drink some Chamomile tea. The great benefit about this herbal remedy is that you can use this as an alternative to medicine. It can help reduce your menstrual cramps. Warmth of Chamomile does relax your muscles that can take away your pain very easily.
- Caffeine increases your menstrual cramps. Avoid caffeine during your period as it can speed up the bleeding as well.
- Use heating pad on you lower abdomen. It will ease the pain.
- Take a walk outdoors that will help alleviate the pain. Walking will keep you feeling more relaxed. If you do not feel doing exercise then walking will be a good alternative and it's as beneficial.
- Ask your husband to massage your back and the areas where your body is aching. It would be a great help.

Remedy

Take liquorices, turmeric and fennel seeds, all same weight and grind them in to a powder. Use 1 tea spoon in the morning and 1 at bed time to get rid of that pain.

If pain still persists take any commercial pain killer and consult the doctor.

21. Migraine

Migraine is just not a headache. It is severe and throbbing pain that can make you unable to function normally at work or even at home. At the same time migraine headaches are very common. They affect women more than men. Without treatment they can occur year after year and even more frequently.

A typical migraine occurs on one side of the head; can be moderate to severe.

It disables a person for daily activities. It also gets intensified by coughing, walking or climbing stairs. In severe cases of migraine a person may vomit, feel nauseated and become very sensitive to light.

Sometimes a sudden depression or exhilaration may cause migraine.

Increased or decreased appetite might cause migraine.

When your sleep is suddenly disrupted it may also cause migraine.

Some migraines are inherited, but most migraines are triggered by diet or by environmental factor.

Alcohol, especially beer and red wine trigger migraine.

Artificial sweeteners like aspartame, Nutrasweet may also trigger migraine.

Processed meats, aged cheeses, perfume or cigarette smoke may also attribute to it.

Sometimes caffeine withdrawal and psychological stress may cause migraine.

Migraine attacks may be prevented by practicing a relaxation technique like deep breathing, meditation, yoga, tai chi.

Regular exercise may help as well. Maintain a regular schedule: Sleep every day for at least seven hours including the weekend. Eat all meals at same time each day.

Do not carry too much heavy bags when travelling. Give yourself enough time to pack.

Do not drink any alcoholic beverage. Some anti-inflammatory herb like feverfew may relieve migraine pain if taken daily. It is available at health Stores. Fish oil supplements might work as well.

If migraine persists see the doctor and use prescribed medication to relieve the pain. You might need more tests and proper neurological evaluation.

22. Minor Burns

- Put cold water on a rag, cloth, or towel and place it on the wound. Hold the cold cloth to the burn for at least 15 minutes to help cool its temperature.
- Apply honey to the wound to help healing and prevent infection. Use papaya on the wound.
- Tea tree oil is a great natural remedy to use when getting rid of burn marks on your feet.
- For razor burn, on a sensitive skin, use Tea tree oil. It is all natural herbal oil with a medicinal healing property. It is often used to soothe and encourage skin irritations.
- Slather mustard on seared skin. After an initial sting, the mustard will relieve the pain and prevent scarring and blistering. It's tested by many people with good results.

23. Motion Sickness

Many people feel sick traveling by air, boat, car or bus. Sometimes motion sickness makes some throw up. Home remedies work wonders. Try some of them if you experience motion sickness:

- Ginger ale or even ginger snaps may help.
- One study found that ginger worked better for motion sickness than anti-nausea medication, and Danish researchers report that ginger helped quell seasickness in susceptible naval cadets better than a placebo.
- Cut a lemon. Sprinkle some salt on one half and suck on it. It will be good to get rid of nausea.
- Just drink lemon water.
- Some people like crystallized ginger. Ginger tea, ginger syrup, or capsules of ginger powder can combat motion sickness and nausea as well.
- A commercial medicine by the name of "jetleg" will also help.

24. Obesity

Obesity is like a disease. It is not easy to control it. When you notice that you are gaining weight that's the time to start controlling it. It needs determination and constant use of certain things and to avoid use of some other things. It is very important to reach your goal of reducing weight. Routinely take your weight. If you put on more than 3 pounds of weight make a schedule to reduce it. Use the following remedies to reduce your weight, and keep up with the plan to maintain certain weight that you feel comfortable with and it makes you look good and healthy.

Use following home remedies:

- Drink I cup of 1% or 2% milk with ½ tea spoon of olive oil added to it every night.
- Avoid greasy food, sweets, rice and potatoes. In six weeks you will see some reduction in your weight.
- Eat between meals. It can also help you lose weight if you choose the right foods. If you are diabetic then eating every few hours can help stabilize blood sugar. Plan your snacks in advance. Add a little protein, Limit snacks to 100 to 200 calories, and make every snack count.

Make a list of healthy snacks: Choose two of them. Stick to your schedule.

- 7-8 walnut halves
- Baby carrots
- 1 cup fat free yogurt
- ½ cup blue berries
- 3 cups of micro-waived popcorns
- 1 small baked potato with 2 tea spoons sour cream, (no butter)
- A small banana will help but take it only some times
- 3 small squares of dark chocolate
- 1 apricot
- 2 celery sticks with table spoon of peanut butter or low fat dip
- 1 grape fruit.
- Avoid eating rice, potatoes or pasta. If you must eat small portions eat on dark color plate. Contrasting colors will

increase awareness of how much you are consuming. Eating food in smaller plate will also make you think you ate a lot.

- Walking 20 minutes every day will also make you reduce some weight.
- Multi-tasking will help. Exercise in front of TV. Water the plants while walking around the house. While on phone walk around.
- As a home remedy in 4 oz of skim milk add ¼ spoon of turmeric powder and drink it either at night or first thing in the morning to lose weight.
- Turmeric is a healthy and inexpensive spice and is not only great for cooking, but it also may help to limit weight gain from a high fat diet. Use it cooking foods.

25. Stress

Modern life is full of hassles, frustrations, and demands. Stress is so common these days that it has become a way of life. A little bit of stress helps some people to perform and get motivated. They do their best under pressure. But constant stress causes chronic fatigue, headaches, a change in eating habits, inability to concentrate and general irritability. In this situation then stress becomes a negative force. These physiological responses of stress trigger adrenaline output. As a result heart pumps faster and breathing rate goes up. Not only that sometimes a person may get so used to it that it becomes normal for him to live under stress.

It's important to learn how to recognize when your stress levels are out of control. You don't notice how much it's affecting you, even as it takes a heavy toll. Stress affects the mind, body, and behavior in many ways, and everyone experiences stress differently.

There are some home remedies to treat stress if it has not reached to the level where normal life is incapacitated. Then relaxation is needed and these home remedies will work. First manage stress by learning how to take charge of your thoughts, emotions, environment, and the way you deal with problems.

Use some home remedies to relax yourself.

It is not easy for everyone these days to indulge in a beauty salon treatment, a massage or facial or join gym. Take a warm bath after the day's work, or household chores using 1 spoon kosher salt or sea salt, 1 spoon baking soda and1 spoon Epsom salt. Soak yourself for at least half hour. You will feel very relaxed.

To give yourself relaxation from anxiety and stress use balm, lavender, passionflower herb, kava root, chamomile, and licorice root.

Do some exercise. Stretch and tap your body. Remember the song 'head and shoulders". Drink green tea.

Prayer is a form of meditation that helps to slow down breathing and brain activity and reduces high blood pressure. Feeling peace, joy and other positive emotions are physiological responses that boost our immune system and reduce arterial inflammation.

Be thankful to God for the good things in your life. Daily gratitude can dramatically decrease stress and give you the feelings of peace and tranquility.

26. Toothache

Toothache is a very nagging pain. It's so difficult to do anything until the pain is relieved.

For immediate relief put a clove on the painful tooth. Clove is antiseptic as well as anesthetic.

Gargle your mouth with lukewarm water and salt many times. Give this about 2 minutes and pain will be gone. It's very affective.

Dab a cotton ball with hydrogen peroxide and rub it over sore gum/tooth area a couple of times. Peroxide will pull some of that infection out of the tooth and its cool liquid on the cotton ball will feel good. You may also rinse your mouth with hydrogen peroxide.

Have some herbal tea, peppermint flavor, boil the water, put a peppermint flavored tea bag in the hot water. Squeeze the tea bag a little and place the hot peppermint tea bag on gums and tooth that are causing pain. After a while take the tea bag out and make sure to swish the tea around a bit when drinking it.

Apply clove oil to the area of pain and rub it on the spot.

Just chew a clove a little and put on the painful tooth.

Clove is anesthetic and will relieve the pain soon.

The juice of the guava leaves cures toothache, swollen gums, and oral ulcers.

Take an Excedrin Migraine pill if the toothache does not go away. Tooth pain is one of the most intense pains there is. For acute pain the only medication that helps is Iboprofin (Motrin) 800mg (but never take on empty stomach). Remember it is a prescription medicine. Go to dentist.

27. Warts

After acne, warts are the most common dermatological complaint. Three out of four people will develop a wart (verruca vulgaris) at some time in their lives.

Warts' treatments are plentiful. If home remedies for warts don't work, you can try over-the-counter wart removers. If your warts still don't disappear, you can turn to treatment by a doctor, who can freeze or cut off the warts.

Home remedies that you may try are:

- Use duct tape to remove warts. It has been shown to work better than freezing them off. Here's how it works: make sure the wart and surrounding skin are clean, then cut a piece of duct tape a bit larger than the wart and press into place. Remove the tape every three days, rub the wart with pumice stone, and repeat until the wart is gone.
- A solution of baking soda and vinegar will cure warts. Keep warts moist with it for 10 minutes. Repeat 3 or 4 times a day. In a week or so warts will disappear.
- A paste of hickory ashes and strong vinegar applied on warts will cure them.
- Rub wart with a slice of raw potato once or twice a day for a few days. Wart will disappear gradually.

Chapter 2

FRESH FRUITS

Fruits should be included in our daily diet to keep us healthy. They are available year round. Only some fruits are seasonal. It's interesting to know about the benefits and the common ailments these fruits can take care of. Make best use of them when they are available. Here is some detailed information about all these fruits (and vegetables in the next chapter) because they are the healthiest foods you can eat with no chemicals and no side effects. They are nature's medicines. And if you buy organically grown fruits the benefits are greater.

1. Apples

Apples are a good source of immune-boosting vitamin C. Apples may actually protect women who get vaginal bleeding from osteoporosis. Apples can also increase the bone density as well as strengthen them. After age 40 actually we should all protect our bones.

- Apples help reduce the effects of Asthma. I have seen young children who suffer from asthma eating apples. A study had shown that many children who eat apples frequently had suffered less from Asthma than those who ate little or hardly any.
- If we eat an apple a day it would rapidly drop our cholesterol rates. This is because of the pectin that we find on the skin of the apples. Do not peel off the skin of the apples. Eat with the skin. An apple a day also keeps dentist away.
- Chances are that the more you eat apples the less you would suffer from breast cancer.
- Pectin found in apples isn't the only ingredient that cures breast and lung cancer it is also a remedy for colon cancer. On

the other hand, pectin can be used to keep a healthy digestive system.

- Fortunately, researchers have also found that apples can greatly reduce liver cancer.
- Apples can protect the brains cells from certain damage which could cause Alzheimer!
- Eat apples as protective source of health and to save yourself from these sicknesses.
- Surprisingly women who eat apples while dieting can lose more weight than women who diet without eating fruit, as some researches show.
- Due to the high amount of flavanoids in apples, those who eat more apples can lower their chances of lung cancer by far. Two of the flavanoids are called quercetin and navinin.
- Apples are good source of iron. When you cut the apple and leave it for some time it start turning brown. This chemical change occurs due to apples having iron in them. An apple a day would be especially good for one who is anemic.

2. Avocado

Avocado as a fruit seems to have no taste. But mixing it with other ingredients it has some good benefits. When available we should use it as part of our diet.

- Avocados are served mixed with white rice, in soups, salads, or on the side of chicken and meat. Avocado slices are frequently added to hamburgers, and hot dogs.
- Avocado can be combined with eggs (in scrambled eggs, tortillas or omelets), and is a key ingredient in California rolls and rolled sushi.
- Avocados are frequently used for milkshakes and occasionally added to ice cream and other desserts in different south Asian and South American countries.
- It is very easy to make a dessert drink of avocados. Just add sugar, milk or water, and pureed avocado and it is ready. For change of taste you may add chocolate syrup. Chilled avocado and milk drink that is sweetened with confectioner's sugar and hinted with orange flower water is also very popular in Southern countries.
- About 75% of an avocado's energy comes from monounsaturated fat as oleic acid.

- It has potential for lowering risk of diabetes mellitus, has antibacterial component and potential anti-cancer activity.
- It may lower blood cholesterol levels.
- The saturated fat is amounting to 14% of total fat in a single serving of avocado. By comparison, edible seeds and nuts have saturated fat content that is approximately 7% of total fat per serving (example, walnuts and almonds).
- Fresh avocado added to a hamburger meal appears to help blood flow in the peripheral arteries.

3. Banana

Have you ever said to someone or a child, "Don't go bananas"? It's because eating a banana a day up-lifts your energy level and facilitates the cross-talk among your brain cells and the effect of mood. Eating a banana lifts brain chemicals like serotonin. Bananas are also rich in potassium. Its deficiency can manifest in a variety of ways, including lethargy and memory problems. Banana does not only keep the dentist away it can keep the therapist away by preventing recurring minor depression. And besides coffee, bananas are our largest dietary source of antioxidants. This necessary nutrient, which is also found in dried apricots, figs, and plums, helps regulate the body's nervous and muscular systems.

Include about four bananas a week in your diet whether sliced over cereal or blended in a smoothie, or just peel it and eat it monkey style. Scientific researches show these benefits of bananas:

- One banana has 11% of the FDA of dietary fiber and only about 108 calories. The fiber in bananas not only keeps digestion regular, but also helps maintain low blood sugar and curbs overeating.
- Studies show that the high amounts of potassium in bananas (over 13% of FDA) can lower one's blood pressure, which in turn lessens the possibility of atherosclerosis, heart attack and stroke. This is very impressive function of the easily available, affordable and likable fruit.
- Along with lowering blood pressure, potassium prevents the weakening of the body's bones. Typical American diets have lot of sodium which can cause the loss of excessive amount of calcium through the urine. The strength and general health of the bones could be threatened. The potassium found in bananas neutralizes the high amounts of sodium in one's diet,

thus allowing for healthy amounts of calcium to remain within the body.

- Bananas also contain high levels of "fructo-oligo-saccharide" (FOS) that promotes calcium absorption. FOS further nourishes healthy bacteria in the colon that manufacture vitamins and digestive enzymes that boost the body's overall ability to absorb nutrients.
- Banana is helpful in diarrhea and in Asian countries it is said that for constipation eat 2 bananas at a time with 2 cardamoms. The high amounts of potassium in bananas can restock electrolytes that are easily depleted when suffering from diarrhea, with potassium being an important electrolyte itself.
- Bananas protect the healthy constitution of the stomach in two ways. Firstly, they trigger the production of mucus in the stomach, which provides a protective barrier against stomach acids. Secondly, bananas possess protease inhibitors, a substance that breaks down bacteria in the stomach that cause ulcers.
- One banana has an impressive 34 % of the FDA of vitamin B6, which serves many important roles in the body's health. For example, the B6 in bananas acts as an anti-inflammatory agent that helps ward off cardiovascular disease, type 2 Diabetes, as well as obesity.

Some home remedies

- You can do a lot more with a banana than just slice it on your cereal.
- Slap a banana peel (the inside part) on an itch caused by a bug bite or poison ivy; this will dial down the inflammation and relieve the itch.
- Just rub the inside part of the peel over your clean face to get the anti-inflammatory and anti-microbial effects.
- Place the inside part of the banana peel on your forehead if suffering from headache.
- If you have leg cramps eat a banana and drink lot of water.

4. Blueberries

Blueberries are perennial flowering plants packed with lots of antioxidants and have a low sugar contents, making them one of the healthiest fruits.

Antioxidants are essential to optimize health by helping to combat the free radicals that can damage cellular structures as well as DNA. Blueberries are therefore ranked in the U.S. diet as having one of the highest antioxidant capacities among all fruits. Not only they are eaten as a fruit, they are used in blueberry muffins, pies and cakes as well.

In U.S. blueberries are second to strawberries in popularity of berries. Blueberry muffins are very popular among children.

Just ½ cup doubles the amount of antioxidants most Americans get in a day.

5.   Cantaloupe

Cantaloupe is the most popular variety of melon in the United States. They are source of vitamin A. Their beta-carotene content can reach levels as high as 3,138 micrograms (per 100 grams of fresh weight). That's about 30 times higher than the beta-carotene content of fresh oranges.

Honey dew is another variety of cantaloupe and is much sweeter and juicier. Diabetic patients should be careful of the intake of this fruit and water melon.

Cantaloupes can be from very small to at least 10 pounds in weight. It is normally eaten as a fresh fruit. But there are various uses of and many varieties of cantaloupe. People use it as a salad, or as a dessert with ice cream or custard. It is also used as a part of mixed fruit serving.

- Cantaloupe has been found to lower risk of metabolic syndrome. Metabolic syndrome is a combination of the medical disorders that, when occur together, increase the risk of developing cardiovascular disease and diabetes.
- In a study involving hundreds of women living and teaching in Tehran, Iran, the lowest risk of metabolic syndrome was found to occur in women who ate the greatest amount, minimum of 12 ounces per day, of fruit. We should include the intake of that much cantaloupe in our daily diet when the fruit is still available. Women have to take care of their health more as these days they have double and in some cases more than double responsibilities.

6.   Cherries

Cherries are an excellent source of potassium, which helps to lower blood pressure by getting rid of the excess sodium in our body. Eating cherries helps keep potassium and sodium in balance, and can prevent hypertension from occurring.

Eating cherries can help you lose weight and stay trim. A cup of cherries is less than 100 calories. Also, these little beauties contain many B-vitamins such as thiamin, riboflavin and vitamin B6; these vitamins are crucial for metabolism and convert nutrients into energy. What could be better than eating cherries to help you stay lean and skinny? Cherries are eaten as fresh fruit in season. Cherries are also used in ice cream, juices and drinks, pies, chocolate and many other things.

Cherries are not only healthy, but they are delicious and versatile. They can be added to everything, eaten raw or cooked down to make a sauce or strained for juice.

A study at the University of Michigan found that a diet that includes a lot of cherries lowers all the overall risk factors for heart disease, including inflammation, body fat, and cholesterol.

- Cherries help in prevention of heart disease.
- These berries can relieve pain of arthritis, gout, and headaches, and ease the symptoms associated with Fibromyalgia Syndrome.
- Cherries have a magnificent taste, sweet or sour. Their taste stands alone but they are also great in desserts or even dried for an afternoon snack.
- Cherries may help fight cancer.
- Cherries help keep you trim.

7.   Coconut

The coconut is a best source of nutritious meat, juice, milk, and oil that for generations has used and nourished populations around the world. It is called "The Tree of Life" in South Asian countries. I know because I was born in India. There people use coconut, all parts of it, for everything. Coconut water is the best thirst quencher. Coconut milk is used in cooking meat, vegetarian and sweet dishes. Fresh coconut is eaten fondly by young and adult alike. Dried coconut, shredded coconut, flaked coconut, ground coconut, and coconut flour, you name it and it is used in one way or the other. Coconut oil is most famous for hair care, skincare and of course for cooking.

Coconut is rich in fiber, vitamins, and minerals. Pacific Islanders consider coconut oil to be the cure for all illness. The coconut palm is so highly valued by them as both a source of food and medicine.

Recently modern medical science has started researching the coconut's amazing healing powers.

The source of the following information is with permission of Dr. Bruce Fife, Director of Coconut Research Center. He mentions it in his article.

"Coconut in Traditional Medicine"

"People from many diverse cultures, languages, religions, and races scattered around the globe have revered the coconut as a valuable source of both food and medicine. Wherever the coconut palm grows the people have learned of its importance as an effective medicine. For thousands of years coconut products have held a respected and valuable place in local folk medicine.

In traditional medicine around the world coconut is used to treat a wide variety of health problems including the following: abscesses, asthma, baldness, bronchitis, bruises, burns, colds, constipation, cough, dropsy, dysentery, earache, fever, flu, gingivitis, gonorrhea, irregular or painful menstruation, jaundice, kidney stones, lice, malnutrition, nausea, rash, scabies, scurvy, skin infections, sore throat, swelling, syphilis, toothache, tuberculosis, tumors, typhoid, ulcers, upset stomach, weakness, and wounds.

He continues to tell us how coconut is treated in modern science for medical purposes and for treatment of many ailments.

Coconut in modern medicine

Modern medical science is now confirming the use of coconut in treating many of the above conditions. Published studies in medical journals show that coconut in one form or another may provide a wide range of health benefits. Some of these are summarized below:

- Kills viruses that cause influenza, herpes, measles, hepatitis C, SARS, AIDS, and other illnesses.
- Kills bacteria that cause ulcers, throat infections, urinary tract infections, gum disease and cavities, pneumonia, and gonorrhea, and other diseases.
- Kills fungi and yeasts that cause candidiasis, ringworm, athlete's foot, thrush, diaper rash, and other infections.
- Expels or kills tapeworms, lice, giardia, and other parasites.
- Provides a nutritional source of quick energy.

- Boosts energy and endurance, enhancing physical and athletic performance.
- Improves digestion and absorption of other nutrients including vitamins, minerals, and amino acids.
- Improves insulin secretion and utilization of blood glucose.
- Relieves stress on pancreas and enzyme systems of the body.
- Reduces symptoms associated with pancreatitis.
- Helps relieve symptoms and reduce health risks associated with diabetes.
- Reduces problems associated with mal-absorption syndrome and cystic fibrosis.
- Improves calcium and magnesium absorption and supports the development of strong bones and teeth.
- Helps protect against osteoporosis.
- Helps relieve symptoms associated with gallbladder disease.
- Relieves symptoms associated with Crohn's disease, ulcerative colitis, and stomach ulcers.
- Improves digestion and bowel function.
- Relieves pain and irritation caused by hemorrhoids.
- Reduces inflammation.
- Supports tissue healing and repair.
- Supports and aids immune system function.
- Helps protect the body from breast, colon, and other cancers.
- Is heart healthy; improves cholesterol ratio reducing risk of heart disease.
- Protects arteries from injury that causes atherosclerosis and thus protects against heart disease.
- Helps prevent periodontal disease and tooth decay.
- Functions as a protective antioxidant.
- Helps to protect the body from harmful free radicals that promote premature aging and degenerative disease.
- Does not deplete the body's antioxidant reserves like other oils do.
- Improves utilization of essential fatty acids and protects them from oxidation.
- Helps relieve symptoms associated with chronic fatigue syndrome.
- Relieves symptoms associated with benign prostatic hyperplasia (prostate enlargement).
- Reduces epileptic seizures.
- Helps protect against kidney disease and bladder infections.
- Dissolves kidney stones.

- Helps prevent liver disease.
- Is lower in calories than all other fats.
- Supports thyroid function.
- Promotes loss of excess weight by increasing metabolic rate.
- Is utilized by the body to produce energy in preference to being stored as body fat like other dietary fats.
- Helps prevent obesity and overweight problems.
- Applied topically helps to form a chemical barrier on the skin to ward of infection.
- Reduces symptoms associated the psoriasis, eczema, and dermatitis.
- Supports the natural chemical balance of the skin.
- Softens skin and helps relieve dryness and flaking.
- Prevents wrinkles, sagging skin, and age spots.
- Promotes healthy looking hair and complexion.
- Provides protection from damaging effects of ultraviolet radiation from the sun.
- Helps control dandruff.
- Does not form harmful by-products when heated to normal cooking temperature like other vegetable oils do.
- Has no harmful or discomforting side effects.
- Is completely non-toxic to humans."

Coconut oil is described as "the healthiest oil on earth." It's the oil that makes it a truly remarkable food and medicine. What makes coconut oil so good?

The difference is in the fat molecule or fatty acids. Coconut oil contains active ingredients that provide brain with ketones needed to improve function in Alzheimer's patients. This is also a natural Candida treatment.

Coconut oil is good for hair care. It makes them grow longer, thicker and shinier. It is also good for skin care. It makes the skin smooth, soft and without blemishes.

Then we have coconut water. Coconut water hydrates the body, and relieves urinary problems. It kills intestinal worms, and breaks kidney stones. Coconut water is antibacterial, and controls vomiting.

Grated coconut is used in candies, chocolates and many Indian sweet dishes. It is also added in lentils and other dishes. Coconut milk is used for cooking meals and sweets.

8. Dates

Allah Almighty mentioned palm trees many times in the Holy Book Quran, and made it the food of the dwellers of Paradise. Dates are one of the world's oldest cultivated and the most nourishing fruits. Sometimes they are called the "Bread of Desert".

Dates can be eaten raw or cooked. Dates can be used into stews, sauces, curries and meat dishes. Dates are delicious either way you eat, whether you serve them with cheese or bake into cookies and cakes. Stuff dates with walnuts or almonds. These make delicious desserts and appetizers. Today, dates are widely-grown in the Arabian Peninsula, Iran, India, Pakistan, Egypt, Iraq, Spain, Italy, and the United States. There are more than 600 varieties of dates.

Before dates ripen they range in color. Ripe dates' color changes to a dark brown. Unripe, full size and crunchy, ripe and soft, and ripe and sun-dried are the 4 stages of the ripening process of dates. For all these stages there are special names Arabs have given them and each is regarded for its unique culinary properties and they are enjoyed eating almost at all stages.

Dates are high in natural sugars like glucose, fructose, and sucrose and make a perfect snack for an immediate burst of energy. Many people around the world use dates for a quick afternoon snack. If you want to increase your weight, or if you are trying to build your muscles, or you have become weak due to a serious medical problem, dates will help you gain weight and they will give you energy.

It was said by the Prophet (peace be upon him) that if you have dates and bread in the house, then you cannot be left hungry. Some health specialists have said that eating one date per day is necessary for a balanced and healthy diet. There are different ways of eating dates. You may mix the paste of the dates with milk or yogurt. Spread the paste and butter on bread and make it even more delicious. The paste is good for both adults and children, especially during a time of recovery from injury or illness.

In Muslim countries or wherever Muslims live, in the month of Ramadan, which is their fasting month, they break their fast by eating dates and water or any home-made drink (water, milk and sugar) according to their cultural traditions. Breaking fast by eating dates is following the tradition of their prophet Mohammad (peace be upon him). It provides basic nutrients to the fasting body and helps the intake of food by the people. When the body begins to absorb the high nutritional value of the dates, feelings of hunger are pacified. The other benefit is that the nervous system can get a lot of help from consuming potassium rich dates. Some health specialists have said that eating one date per day is necessary for a balanced and healthy diet.

"One who starts the morning every day with the date of Ajwa, poison and magic will not affect him that day till the night. Another narrator mentioned seven dates of Ajwa." Bukhari (5768)

Ajwa is a variety of dates especially grown in Medina, Saudi Arabia.

They are extremely nutritious and contain more natural sugar than any other fruit. Dates contain protein, Vitamin A, and some of the B vitamins, potassium, oil, calcium, sulfur, iron, phosphorous, manganese, copper and magnesium. All of them are necessary for maintaining good health. Seven dates weigh approximately 100 grams which provides a sufficient intake of a wide variety of minerals, salts and vitamins for the body.

Dates have a high mineral content, but they have an impressive level of iron which makes them a perfect dietary supplement for anemic patients. Use of dates increases energy and strength, and decreases feelings of fatigue and sluggishness. Drinking dates juice could be used in the treatment of sore throat, various types of fever and common cold.

Dates can be used for many common ailments such as constipation, intestinal disorders, heart problems, anemia, sexual dysfunction, diarrhea, abdominal cancer, and many other conditions. Dates are a laxative food. People suffering from constipation should eat dates. Soak them in water over night then eat the soaked dates in the morning. Because of the high levels of soluble fiber, dates promote healthy bowel movements.

The significant amounts of minerals found in dates make it a super food for strengthening bones and fighting off painful and debilitating diseases like osteoporosis. Dates contain selenium, manganese, copper, and magnesium, all of which are integral to healthy bone development and strength, particularly as people begin to age and their bones gradually weaken. So, eat your dates and give a boost to your bones!

The American Cancer Society recommends an intake of 20-35 grams of dietary fiber per day, which can be supplied through dates. Vitamin A and vitamin K in dates protect eyes against blindness.

Actually dates are a wholesome meal in themselves. They are also good source of maintaining health and protecting body from various ailments.

9. Grapefruit

Grapefruit is a citrus fruit. In the latter part of the 19th century grapefruit began to be cultivated commercially. It has a high level of vitamin C and contains high amount of enzymes and potassium that helps in weight loss by burning fat in the body.

Its high level of vitamin C helps fight the common cold and flu. It aids bowel movements and promotes digestion. Its low contents in sodium and calories are also an excellent aid for reducing weight. High (90 percent) water content helps increase metabolism. One half of a grapefruit contains only 74 calories, which makes it a favorable choice for people who want to go on diet to reduce their weight. It is an aid in repairing DNA damage as well. DNA repair can help prevent cancer because of its function in reducing mutations in cells.

As a result of a joint study undertaken by scientists from the University of California at Los Angeles and Zhongshan University in China, Naringenin, a compound found in grapefruit, was found to be helpful in repairing damaged DNA material in prostate cancer cells.

Grapefruit can also helpful in reducing cholesterol. One grapefruit a day lowers bad cholesterol significantly.

Grapefruit juice is citric and has natural sugars. It also boosts immune system. It is rich in folic acid and potassium.

10. Grapes

Grapes are one of the most delicious fruits. They are rich sources of vitamins A, C, B6 and Folate. They are also full of essential minerals like potassium, calcium, iron, phosphorus, magnesium and selenium. Grapes contain flavonoids that are very powerful antioxidants, which can reduce the damage caused by free radicals and slow down ageing. Grapes play an important role in ensuring a healthy and robust life.

Grapes if used regularly treat constipation, indigestion, fatigue, kidney disorders, macular degeneration and prevention of cataract.

They are good for Asthma, heart diseases, breast cancer, and Alzheimer's disease. They have anti-bacterial activity and anti-cancer properties.

Thus, grapes play a pivotal role in preventing innumerable health disorders and can be used as home based remedies for several ailments. Grapes also control blood cholesterol.

Dried grapes, known as raisins, are extremely nutritious and help in many disorders including constipation, acidosis, anemia, fever, sexual weakness and help in gaining weight and eye care. Dried grapes or raisins may be soaked overnight and eaten in the morning along the water they are soaked in, for constipation, anemia, and eye care. Because of being beneficial for health raisins are used in baking cookies and candies, and in many desserts. They are even used in Afghani rice dishes, in Indo-Pakistani desserts and other sweet dishes. They are part of the mixed dried fruits. They are used in many cereals. Raisins also make a good snack for children and adults alike. They are correctly called "nature's candies".

11. Guava

Guava is very common in Asian countries. It's a seasonal tropical fruit, and is a real storehouse of nutrients. It is said that "a few guavas in the season keep the doctor away for the whole year" in the Indian Subcontinent and places where guavas grow. It is one of the least sprayed fruit. It is mostly organic. Those who want to lose weight should eat guavas because they have no cholesterol and less digestible carbohydrates. Guava is also very filling and satisfies appetite very easily. Guava has far lesser amounts of sugars as compared to apple, orange, grapes, and other fruits. Just have a medium sized guava in the lunch and you will not feel hungry till evening.

Eating a guava makes your gums feel tighter and fresh after you chew a raw guava. It is good remedy for diarrhea. As it has anti-bacterial and disinfectant, it helps cure dysentery. In third world countries it is a common disease. It is misunderstood as diarrhea. Guava is also beneficial in gastroenteritis. Potassium in guava also strengthens and tones up the digestive system and disinfects it. Proper digestion and more importantly, proper excretion ensures our total health. Constipation and improper digestion cause many other ailments in human body.

Juice of raw and immature guavas or decoction of guava-leaves is very helpful in giving relief in cough and cold by loosening cough, reducing mucus, disinfecting the respiratory tract, throat and lungs and inhibiting microbial activity due to its astringent properties. In some parts of India roasted ripe guava is used as a remedy against extreme cases of cough, cold, and congestion.

Guava, being very rich in fiber and hypoglycemic in nature, helps reduce blood pressure, helps reduce cholesterol, prevents blood from thickening, and maintains fluidity of blood.

Guavas and their leaves are very useful in treating skin texture. This is chiefly due to the abundance of astringents in it and in leaves. You can benefit from it by eating the fruits or by washing your skin with the decoction of its immature fruits and leaves. It will tone up and tighten the loosened skin, and will keep your skin glowing and free from aging, wrinkles and other disorders. Vitamin E contents in guava help maintain healthy skin through its antioxidant properties.

Vitamin C is the only remedy to its deficiency which causes scurvy. Guava has concentration of Vitamin C, more than orange or any other fruit. It helps to prevent the viral infections like cold and cough. Guava helps control diabetes. The juice of the leaves cures toothache, swollen gums & oral ulcers. It heals wounds when applied externally. It heals convulsions, epilepsy, bacterial infections and being a rich source of dietary fiber, it helps to cure constipation.

Magnesium in guavas helps to relax the nerves and muscles in the body. Guava is packed with vitamins and minerals that help to keep the skin healthy and fresh Guavas are very good sources of vitamin A, the nutrient best known for preserving and improving eyesight.

If you do not want to eat banana, eat a guava. They both have same amount of potassium. Potassium helps in regulating blood pressure by reversing the role of sodium in unbalancing normal blood pressure.

Guava is a cholesterol free fruit. It satisfies and keeps the stomach free from hunger for a long time. It assists in weight reduction. Guava if available should be consumed regularly if you want to avoid heart attack.

12. Kiwi Fruit

Kiwi fruit is the most nutrient-rich of the top 26 fruits consumed in the world today. It also has the highest density of any fruit for vitamin C and magnesium limited mineral in the food supply of most affluent countries and a nutrient important for cardiovascular health.

Banana, citrus fruits and Kiwi are among the top three low-sodium, and high-potassium fruits, but kiwifruit ranks number one. It has more potassium than a banana or any citrus fruit.

Kiwi fruit is excellent source of vitamin C. It has dietary fiber. Vitamin C helps make the skin softer and more resilient. It helps make the skin flexible and wrinkle free. According to FDA kiwifruit would also be a good source of vitamin E and potassium. The FDA considers kiwifruit a good source of vitamin E, crucial for a healthy heart. Kiwifruit is low fat and contains no cholesterol, rich in many Vitamins, flavonoids and minerals and a good amount of beta-carotene.

This fruit may contain an anti-mutagenic component, helping to prevent the mutations of genes that may initiate the cancer process.

Inositol, a sugar alcohol naturally occurring, is also found in kiwifruit, and because of its function as a precursor of an intracellular second messenger system, Kiwi can be beneficial in the treatment of depression. Inositol may play a positive role in regulating diabetes as well. Inositol supplements may be bought from pharmacies or health stores and be taken to improve diabetic neuropathy.

Kiwifruit contains lot of beta carotenes, Lutein, and xanthophylls, and antioxidants, including vitamins C and E. The excellent complement of antioxidants in kiwifruit may help prevent the oxidation of the good cholesterol (HDLs).

Two amino acids, arginine and glutamate, are found in Kiwi fruit. Arginine may help promote an increase in arteriolar dilation, working as a vasodilator and improving blood flow. That is important for heart health.

Kiwifruit contains magnesium at 6% DV. Magnesium is thought to be in short supply in the diets of affluent countries. Poor magnesium status is associated with heart disease, myocardial infarction and hypertension. Pectin contained in this fruit has been shown to lower cholesterol.

The sodium-to-potassium is extremely favorable in kiwifruit which is critical for heart health. Kiwifruit could be an immune booster due to its extremely high vitamin C content. Kiwifruit contains a wide range of minerals (electrolytes) essential for replenishing those lost during exercise, in hot weather, due to high fever. It is also a naturally significant source of electrolytes for a pre-workout regimen as well.

Kiwifruit contains a relatively high level of serotonin. Serotonin causes a calming effect in most cases.

Several anti-aging skin care products contain kiwi fruit extracts to help diminish fine lines and wrinkles.

Kiwi fruit helps in healing cuts and bruises by producing extra collagen needed. It also helps fight against skin dryness and flakiness. It can treat acne scars, hyper-pigmentation, and skin discoloration.

13. Lemon

Lemon is a super food which is full of health and cosmetics benefits. Lemon is a delicious, juicy, citrus fruit that is easily available in any supermarket. Benefits of lemon have been known for centuries. Lemon is rich in vitamins that are necessary for body. Lemon is the source of vitamin C, magnesium, copper, iron, zinc, manganese, potassium and phosphorus.

Drinking lemon water has many benefits. It is a natural energizer. It hydrates and oxygenates the body so it feels revitalized and refreshed. It also boosts immune system, balances pH, decreases wrinkles and blemishes. Lemon water also cures throat infections, reduces fever, purifies blood, flushes out unwanted material and is excellent source of weight loss. It also helps in relieving tooth pain.

The most important benefit of lemon is that it makes you fresh especially in summers. Lemonade is a cherished household drink that makes people refresh and healthy. Indeed it can rejuvenate you after a tiring day. People also like to drink lemon tea. Lemons have been a quite effective home remedy for a many of health problems. Lemon is a strong antibacterial and antiviral agent. It acts as a liver cleanser and aids in weight loss. It promotes immunity, sleep and fight infection. Lemon drink is helpful in removing fatigue, exhaustion, dizziness, anxiety, nervousness and tension. It is also helpful in increasing alertness and concentration.

Lemon juice is a good remedy in fever, cold or flu. It assists in breaking fever by increasing perspiration. Lemon contains citric acid which is effective in treating acne. The vitamin C in lemon is vital for healthy glowing skin while its alkaline nature kills some types of bacteria known to cause acne. After you have squeezed the juice out of half a lemon turn it inside out and give your face and nose a good scrub with it. It will treat your oily skin and work on pimples and acne.

Lemon juice with turmeric powder and honey is s good paste to treat oily skin and reduce pimples, blackheads and acne.

Lemon juice can also be applied to stop sun burn.

Use lemon juice on your hair before shower to give your hair a natural shine. It is also a good remedy for dandruff. Lemon acts as blood purifier. It is helpful in treating diseases like malaria and cholera. It helps to flush bacteria and toxins out of body. If you are an asthma patient then you should take one tablespoon lemon juice one hour before every meal.

The freshly squeezed lemon juice applied on aching tooth can reduce toothache. When massaged on gums, it cures all wounds of gums and stops gum bleeding. Its use kills bad smell.

Massaging lemon on nails is very beneficial for making your nails shining. It is very useful in removing stains, using it in the wash and making clothes smell fresh. In many dish washing liquids lemon is used for fresh smell. Many foods are prepared with lemon juice added to them. Simply use lemon because it is a natural product with no chemical additives.

Lemon peel has its own benefits. First of all lemon peel contains 5 to 10 times more vitamins than the lemon juice itself. It is good for oral hygiene and hygiene, bone health, internal parasites and worms, weight loss, cancer, bacterial infections and fungi. Lemon peel can also be used for regulating blood pressure, as antidepressant and to keep out insects.

14. Mango

Mango is called "The king of the fruits," in many tropical countries and is one of the most popular, nutritionally rich fruits with unique flavor, fragrance, taste, and health promoting qualities. Mango is often labeled as one of the "super fruits."

Mango is one of the delicious seasonal fruits that grow in the tropical countries. Fresh mango season starts in April and lasts until August. Its flavor is pleasant and rich, and tastes sweet with mild tartness. A high-quality mango fruit contains no or very little fiber and is sweet. Good quality mango does not have sour taste. Mango can be enjoyed all alone without any additions.

- Fresh mango cubes are a great addition to fruit salads.
- Mango juice with ice cubes is a popular, delicious drink.
- Mango fruit juice blended with milk as "mango-milk shake" or mango lassi with yogurt.
- Mango fruit is also used to prepare jam, ice cream and in candy industries.
- The unripe, raw, green mango has been used in the preparation of pickles.
- The raw mango is used in making, jam (marmalade), and chutney in the Asian countries.
- Mango preserves are made with ripe mangoes.
- Raw mango slices may be added to some vegetarian dishes in place of lemon.
- A raw mango slice may be added to soups to give it a little tart taste.
- Mangoes may be peeled, sliced and be frozen for off season use.

Long time ago when I was in India I had read a small booklet about the health benefits of mango. It had listed one hundred and one benefits. I do not remember all of them but some stayed in my memory:

- It is blood purifier.
- It is laxative.
- It helps producing red blood cells.
- Mango lassi (mango milk/yogurt shake) is very satisfying and digestive when drank at meals.
- It is good for skin.
- Its use opens clogged pores.
- It eliminates pimples.
- It promotes good eyesight and prevents night blindness and dry eyes.
- It improves sex life.
- The fiber in mangos also helps digestion.
- Drinking mango drink (mango juice water and sugar) is a good remedy for heat stroke.
- It is good during pregnancy.

But now we have scientific research on the health benefits of mango. This is what the research says about it:

- Mango is rich in pre-biotic dietary fiber, vitamins, minerals, and poly-phenolic flavonoid antioxidant compounds.
- According to new research study, mango may be helpful in protecting against colon, breast, leukemia and prostate cancers.
- Fresh mango is a good source of potassium. 100 g fruit provides 156 mg of potassium while just 2 mg of sodium. Potassium is an important component of cell and body fluids that helps controlling heart rate and blood pressure.
- It is also a very good source of vitamin-B6 (pyridoxine) and vitamin-E.
- Mango is an excellent source of Vitamin-A and flavonoids like beta-carotene, alpha-carotene, and beta-cryptoxanthin.
- Vitamin C helps the body develop resistance against infectious agents and scavenge harmful oxygen-free radicals. Vitamin B-6 is required for GABA hormone production within the brain.
- Further, mango composes moderate amounts of copper. Copper is a co-factor for many vital enzymes. Copper is also required for the production of red blood cells.
- Additionally, mango peel is also rich in the pigment antioxidants like carotenoids and polyphenols.

15. Oranges

Oranges are one of the most popular and favorite fruits in the world. They taste delicious and sour, and contain several vitamins. Vitamins protect our body from many harmful diseases and illnesses while having a number of cures.

- Oranges are beneficial incurring Asthma.
- Eating oranges also prevents forming kidney stones.
- They are helpful in lowering cholesterol level.
- Oranges may help in controlling high blood pressure.
- Continuous use of oranges may prevent one from developing diabetes.
- Oranges help your stomach stimulate digestive juices to relieve the stiffness of your bowels?
- Eating the flesh of an orange would be good for your dieting as it contains 3.1 grams of fiber. It is recommended to take in 25-35 grams of fiber daily.
- Orange keeps your skin young and moisturized.
- Another health benefit of oranges is that there is a powerful antioxidant called Beta-carotene which protects skin cells from getting damaged.
- Use the orange peel for other health benefits! Orange peels are useful for exfoliating facial scrub.
- Orange peel oil bath is healthy for the skin.
- Orange zest into your diet can give you an extra 3 grams of fiber. Rest of the fiber can be compensated from other fruits and vegetables in our diet.
- Orange zest can flavor your cooking recipes.
- Orange peels can be used to keep cats, ants and slugs away from your garden.
- Orange peels can kindle your house fire.
- Orange peel is a deodorizer.
- Rubbing fresh orange peel can repel mosquitoes.
- Taking one or two oranges at bedtime and again on rising in the morning is an excellent way of stimulating the bowels.

16. Papaya

Papaya is a delicious fruit to eat. Papaya can be eaten as a fruit, a smoothie or even a milkshake. Papaya is excellent for the human body.

- Green papaya is used for tenderizing meat and other proteins. It is now included as a component in powdered meat tenderizers. Its ability to break down tough meat fibers was used for thousands of years by indigenous Americans.
- Eating papaya as a ripe fruit helps digest food. It will relieve the constipation and make the bowel movement easy.
- Papaya is low in calories and high in nutritive value. It is an excellent food for those on a diet.
- Papaya contains natural fiber, carotene, vitamin C and essential minerals. Papayas also contain enzymes like arginine and carpain.
- Papaya lowers cholesterol levels. When cholesterol in the body gets oxidized, it can lead to heart-attacks. Papaya supports cardiovascular system.
- Regularly consuming papaya helps to relieve moving sickness and nausea.
- Papaya has anti-inflammatory properties that helps reducing arthritis pain, edema and osteoporosis pain.
- If you use of papaya regularly it will increase energy, and aid in weight loss. Papaya also boosts the immune system.
- The anti-oxidants in papaya also help in controlling premature ageing, which helps to give a young look.
- Papaya is used in many skin lightening creams. Many of the lotions or creams which are used to make the face lighter or fairer contain papaya as an ingredient.
- Papaya also helps in getting rid of acne.
- Papaya prevents cataract formation.
- Use raw papaya as medicine to help in reducing menstrual irregularities and to ease the condition by promoting natural flow of menstruation.

17. Peaches

Peaches are a seasonal fruit. But you can buy canned, frozen, and dried peaches from the markets any time of the year and enjoy them.

Peaches originated in China and were introduced to California by Spanish missionaries in the 1700s. Today they are grown in 36 U.S. states. Although Georgia is called the Peach State, California produces 99% of all cling peaches. Peaches and nectarines belong to same family and are best stored at temperatures of 0°C (32°F) and high-humidity. They are highly perishable, and should be consumed as soon as you buy them.

Some people might be allergic or show some intolerance to this fruit. It is a relatively common form of hypersensitivity to proteins that are found in peaches.

Jams, jellies, and preserves are made with peaches, and peaches are used for filling for desserts cakes and custard. They are used as an ingredient in many other dishes.

Peaches are high in fiber and in Vitamins A, C, and E. They contain calcium that most of the fruits do not. They can help ease dry coughs and relieve constipation.

One medium peach provides only about 50 calories.

Ripe peaches give aroma and some softness so buy them ripe and enjoy them soon.

18. Pears

The pear is a sweet fruit and is related to the apple. Pears are excellent source of water-soluble fiber. They contain vitamins A, B1, B2, C, E, folic acid and niacin. It is also rich in copper, phosphorus and potassium, with lesser amounts of calcium, chlorine, iron, magnesium, sodium and sulfur.

Pear juice is safe to be introduced to infants as it is mild and healthful.

The fruit and its juice both are natural source of energy due largely to having high amounts of fructose and glucose.

The juice is excellent in relieving fever. Best way to bring a fever down quickly is by drinking a big glass of pear juice.

Drink pear juice when you feel a cold coming. It is immune booster. The anti-oxidant nutrients in pears build up your immune system.

Drink pear juice to help clear the phlegm. The summer heat may cause children and some adults to have shortness of breath with excessive phlegm. Juice will help clear it.

Drinking pear juice regularly helps regulate bowel movements because the pectin in pears is diuretic and has a mild laxative effect.

Pear juice is anti-inflammatory and helps relieve pain in various inflammatory conditions.

Pears have anti-oxidant and anti-carcinogen glutathione which help prevent high blood pressure and stroke.

The high vitamin C and copper content act as good anti-oxidants that protect cells from damages by free radicals.

The high content of pectin in pears makes it very useful in helping to lower cholesterol levels.

The high content of folic acid prevents neural tube defects in infants.

Chinese pears

The pears are in season during the summer for a reason. Drinking pear juice every morning and night helps to cool your body down during this time. It nourishes the throat and helps prevent throat problems.

Boil two Chinese pear juice with some raw honey and drink warm. This is extremely healing for the throat and the vocal cord. Good for singers, teachers, speakers etc.

19. Pineapple

Pineapple is a remarkable fruit. It is lush, sweet and has exotic flavor. It may be one of the most healthful foods available today.

Pineapple is valuable for easing indigestion, arthritis or sinusitis.

The juice helps get rid of intestinal worms.

Pineapple is high in manganese, a mineral that is critical to development of strong bones and connective tissue. One-half cup of pineapple chunks contains 11g of carbs. A cup of fresh pineapple will give you nearly 75% of the recommended daily amount.

Pineapples contain bromelain, a rich source of enzymes that aids digestion, speeds up wound healing, and reduces inflammation. They're also an excellent source of mineral manganese, which is necessary for healthy skin, bone and cartilage formation, and glucose tolerance.

It is particularly helpful to older adults, whose bones tend to become brittle with age.

Pineapple is known to be a digestive aid. It helps the body digest proteins more efficiently. Pineapple prevents blood clot development. This makes it a valuable dietary addition for someone who may be at risk for blood clots.

For morning sickness fresh pineapple juice is the best remedy. It really works! The fresh juice discourages dental plaque growth.

20. Pomegranate

Pomegranate is one of the oldest known fruits. It is mentioned in writings and artifacts of many cultures and religions. It is mentioned in Quran as fruit of Paradise. Pomegranate (punica granatum) is an original native of Iran. This fruit is nutrient dense, antioxidant rich and has been revered as a symbol of health, fertility and eternal life.

It is rich in antioxidants that can keep bad LDL cholesterol from oxidizing (American Journal of Clinical Nutrition, May 2000). In addition, pomegranate juice, like aspirin, can help keep blood platelets from clumping together to form unwanted clots. More recent research has found that eight ounces of pomegranate juice daily for three months improved the amount of oxygen getting to the heart muscle of patients with coronary heart disease (American Journal of the College of Cardiology, Sept. 2005).

Drinking 1.7 ounces of pomegranate juice per day lowered blood pressure by as much as 5 percent. Adding pomegranate juice to your daily routine may be a safe and delicious way to reduce your blood pressure. A glass of pomegranate juice has more antioxidants than red wine, green tea, blueberries, and cranberries.

Pomegranate juice acts as an enzyme inhibitor which may prevent cartilage deterioration.

Like most fruits, pomegranates contain plenty of vitamins and fiber. The antibacterial compounds found in pomegranate juice may be a natural way to prevent dental plaque.

Pomegranate juice has shown promise in early studies for its blood pressure lowering effects.

The Mayo Clinic says, "Pomegranate juice is generally safe to drink. Most studies have used a daily intake of 1.5 ounces of pomegranate juice with no significant side effects."

Try tossing the seeds on a salad for a brilliantly colorful, crunchy, and nutritious addition.

21. Strawberries

Strawberries are liked by children and adults alike. Their brilliant red color attracts every one which stimulates the burning of stored fat. They are seasonal and are at their peak from April through July. Strawberries are ranked 4th among all fruits If you're not already a fan of strawberries, you should be. Not only are they juicy, summery and delicious, they're called a super food too.

Their unique *phenol* content makes them heart protective, anti-cancer, and anti-inflammatory.

They are rich in B-complex group of vitamins.

They are a good source of Vitamin C, manganese, fiber, folate, magnesium, copper, and Vitamins B5 and B6.

- The red coloring contains anthocyanins; they stimulate the burning of stored fat.
- The anthocyanins boost short-term memory by 100 % in eight weeks.—The Journal of Agricultural and Food Chemistry.
- One cup of strawberries contains only 49 calories.
- They lower blood levels of C-reactive protein (CRP) which is a signal of inflammation in the body.
- Flavonoids are responsible for the color and flavor of strawberries have been found to help.
- Strawberries contain potassium, vitamin K, and magnesium which are important for eyes and bone health.
- Studies indicate the potential of freeze-dried strawberry powder for preventing human oesophageal cancer.
- Strawberries are filled with biotin, which helps build strong hair and nails. Also contains the antioxidant ellagic acid, which protects the elastic fibers in our skin to prevent sagging.
- The compound nitrate found in strawberries promotes blood flow and oxygen in our body helps with weight loss.
- Eating three or more servings of fruit like strawberries may lower the risk of macular degeneration.—Study in Archives of Ophthalmology.

22. Watermelon

Watermelons are related to cantaloupes, squash, and pumpkins, and originated in Africa. The ancient Egyptians loved watermelons, and even placed them on the tombs of kings. They were brought to China as early as the 10th century, then to the New World in the 1500s.

They are high in Vitamins C, A, B1, and B6. A cup of watermelon contains only about 48 calories. That's because the fruit is 92% water. It is the ideal as a thirst quencher. It is sweet enough to be dessert and good enough for our health as well. It's rich in vitamins and minerals, but low in calories. It soothes sore muscles.

According to a new study in the Journal of Agricultural Food and Chemistry, drinking watermelon juice before a hard workout helped reduce athletes' heart rate and next-day muscle soreness. That's because watermelon is rich in an amino acid called L-citrulline, which the body converts to L-arginine, an essential amino acid that helps relax blood vessels and improve circulation.

Besides tasting great it is low in calories because watermelon is mostly water.

It is an excellent source of Vitamin C which is a major antioxidant.

It has a high beta carotene concentration that offers a fair amount of vitamin A.

Both beta carotene with vitamin A help support good eyesight and prevent glaucoma.

When buying a whole watermelon check that one side of the melon should have an area that is different in color from the rest of the rind. This underbelly shows where the melon rested on the ground until ripe. If this lighter area is missing, the melon may have been harvested prematurely, making it inferior in taste, texture, and juiciness.

Chapter 3

VEGETABLES

1. Bitter Melon

Bitter melon is actually a member of the squash family and resembles a cucumber with bumpy skin. It is bitter in taste. Each bitter melon plant bears separate yellow male and female flowers. As the fruit ripens, the flesh becomes tougher and bitter. But Chinese bitter melon does not taste so bitter.

Bitter melon is used mostly in Asian and Indian cooking. Bitter melon is generally consumed cooked in the green stage. In Chinese cooking, bitter melon is typically stir-fried, or used in soups. Bitter melon tea is also available. In Indian cuisine, bitter melon is stuffed with spices and with or without ground meat and cooked in oil. It is also prepared with curry. Sometimes the spiky part of the skin is scraped and bitter melon is washed with salt and hot water to take off some of the bitterness.

Boiled bitter melon extracts show anti-oxidant activities. It is believed that its strong anti-oxidative activity allows the variety of health benefits of bitter melon.

Bitter melon may also have benefits of lipid-lowering activities.

The results of a study have clearly shown that that bitter melon exhibited a potent liver triglyceride-lowering activity.

Bitter melon is considered to lower blood sugar as it has hypoglycemic properties. Grind and take out the juice and drinking it twice a day will help lower blood sugar. Just consuming bitter melon cooked in variety of ways will also help.

Slice bitter melon and let stand for 30 minutes, drain the juice in a cup. Add some salt and quarter spoon of lemon to cut down the bitter taste and take a spoon full before meals. It will also help lower blood sugar.

It is very important to monitor your blood sugar level to determine if it is helping or not. If not you may try something else. Continue with your prescription medicine.

2. Broccoli

Broccoli is an edible green plant in *the* cabbage family, whose large flower head is used as a vegetable. Broccoli is often boiled or steamed but may be eaten raw. Since the Roman Empire, broccoli has been considered a uniquely valuable food among Italians. It was introduced in USA in 1920s.

Broccoli is low in Saturated Fat, and very low in Cholesterol. It is also a good source of Protein, Thiamin, Pantothenic Acid, Calcium, Iron, Magnesium and Phosphorus, and a very good source of Dietary Fiber, Vitamin A, Vitamin C, Vitamin E, Vitamin K, Riboflavin, Vitamin B6, Folate, Potassium and Manganese.

Broccoli is high in vitamin C and dietary fiber; it also contains multiple nutrients with potent anti-cancer properties. The fiber-related components in broccoli do a better job of binding together with bile acids in your digestive tract when they've been steamed, and the result is a lowering of your cholesterol levels. Raw broccoli still has cholesterol-lowering ability—just not as much.

Boiling broccoli reduces the levels of suspected anti-carcinogenic compounds, besides it becomes soft and mushy, loses its taste and flavor. It is best to steam it or microwave it. You may stir-fry it as well and it will have no significant effect on its compounds. Steaming broccoli only for 5 minutes will preserve all nutrients.

Broccoli has a strong, positive impact on our body's detoxification system is an important aspect of liver metabolism. Broccoli may help us solve our vitamin D deficiency that many people suffer from. Broccoli has strong combination of vitamin A and vitamin K. Broccoli may be an ideal food to include in the diet for supplementing vitamin D.

It provides significant amounts of the lutein and zeaxanthin carotenoids. Lutein in broccoli is good for eyes.

Broccoli sprouts contain highly concentrated levels of these compounds as well as the many vitamins and nutrients that make broccoli such a healthy food. Some of the properties of broccoli have cancer-fighting qualities.

Broccoli is detoxicating in nature and is an important aspect of liver metabolism.

Scientific Researches on Broccoli

Research shows that three-day-old broccoli sprouts have the most potent concentration of cancer fighting compounds.

Sulforaphane in broccoli may inhibit the growth of breast cancer stem cells while helping the liver to oust harmful toxins and carcinogens from the body.

Researchers at John Hopkins found that glucoraphanin, the precursor to sulforphane, is found at highly concentrated levels in broccoli sprouts. Broccoli is touted for its high levels of vitamin C and other great antioxidant benefits. Studies at Johns Hopkins University showed that broccoli sprouts produced 20-50 times more cancer fighting antioxidant activity than broccoli heads.

A study at Ulster University showed that eating around 100 grams of sprouted vegetables every day protects against DNA damage, which is commonly associated with cancer risk.

One study fed rats extracts of broccoli sprouts while exposing them to harmful carcinogens. Those fed the sprout extract developed fewer mammary tumors, smaller tumors, and at slower rates than those not fed the extracts.

3.   Carrots

Carrots are naturally sweet, delicious and crunchy, tasty and highly nutritious, and are healthy additions in our diet. Carrots vary widely in color and shape depending on the cultivar types. They are winter season crops in many parts of Asia and are dark saffron color. In Europe and USA they are orange in color. Both children and adults like carrots because they are sweet tasty and crunchy in texture.

Carrots can even help clean your teeth, and is the best way to keep your mouth clean after meals. They act as natural abrasives that help in eliminating the plague from the teeth and gums. They also trigger a lot of saliva, which helps to scrub away stains on your teeth. Minerals in carrots help to kill germs in the mouth and prevent tooth damage.

Carrot has strong cleansing properties that are effective in detoxifying the liver. They are very effective for acne that is caused by toxins from the blood. Regular consumption of carrots reduces cholesterol levels. Soluble fiber in carrots can help lower blood cholesterol levels by binding with and removing bile acids, cholesterol triggers would be pulled out from the bloodstream to make more bile acids.

Carrots are really an amazing vegetable. There are many benefits of carrots and they are easy to add to your diet without much extra preparation. Carrots are a great source of fiber, which is important for keeping the digestive system running properly. It also helps to keep you feeling full. If you want to go on diet carrots will make you eat less. Carrots are high in nutrition and low in calories, that means that you can fill your stomach without eating too many calories. Additionally, carrots help improve the function of the metabolism because they contains nicotine acid to break down the lipids and fats that are present within the body.

Before using carrots for anything first wash them thoroughly. Then trim both ends and gently scrape off outer skin and smaller hairy roots. Now carrots are ready to be used in any recipe.

In South Asia, a delicious sweet dish called "gaajar ka halwa" is prepared using grated carrot. They are boiled in milk till they are very tender then butter and sugar are added to it. Keep stirring it until all the milk is absorbed and the butter is separating from carrots, then it is ready. Add almonds, cashews and pistachio and mix them well. Garnish "halwa" with all those nuts as well. It makes a very rich sweet dish. Gaajar means carrot.

There is another very popular dish called "gajarbhat". It is made with grated carrots, a small amount of rice, milk and sugar. All ingredients are put together in a heavy pot. After bringing it to boil on high heat bring the flame to medium low and let it simmer for atleast one hour. Stir occasionally. When carrots and rice are very soft and thickened it is ready. It is almost like a pudding. It is very delicious.

Carrots are used in the preparation of cakes, tart, pudding, soups, broth, etc.

They are also used in the preparation of healthy baby-foods.

Carrots are cooked with other vegetables like green beans, potato, peas in many recipes either stewed, in curry, or stir fried.

Carrots can be boiled. Boiling them in water for few minutes enriches their flavor and enhances the bioavailability of nutrients.

Scientific Research on Carrots

Carrots are a good source of vitamin A, vitamin B1, vitamin B2, vitamin B6, vitamin K, vitamin C, biotin, fiber, potassium and thiamine, pantothenic acid, and a compound called poly-acetylene antioxidant falcarinol.

The retina of the eye needs vitamin A to function, lack of vitamin A causes night blindness. Carrots are rich in beta-carotene, a substance which converted into vitamin A in the liver. In the retina, vitamin A is transformed into a purple pigment that is necessary for night vision. In addition, beta-carotene help protect against macular degeneration and the development of senile cataracts. The vitamin A and other nutrients contained in carrot efficiently nourish the skin prevent dry skin and other skin blemishes. The vitamin A in carrots helps the skin by helping to get rid of damaged cells and regenerating new ones. A study found that people who eat most Beta-carotene had 40 percent lower risk of macular degeneration than those who consumed little. Vitamin A also keeps the skin protected from harmful UV rays, retards aging, prevents acne, helps dry skin, and improves the complexion.

Carrot is also useful for treating uneven skin tones due to pigmentation. Carrots contain a lot of beta-carotene, which serves as an antioxidant that helps the body to fight against free radicals. It also help slows down the aging of cells and various negative effect associated with aging.

According to research from Harvard University, people who ate more than six carrots a week are much less likely to suffer a stroke than those who ate only one carrot a month or more.

Eating carrots may help lower the risk of breast cancer, lung cancer and colon cancer. Recently, researchers have isolated a compound called falcarinol in carrots that may be largely responsible for anti-cancer benefits. Falcarinol is a natural pesticide found in carrots that protects roots from fungal diseases. The high levels of antioxidants in carrots help to lower the risk of cancer. Studies have found that carrots may help to prevent three of the most common types of cancer: breast, lung, and colon cancer. They are one of the only food sources of falcarinol, a natural pesticide and fatty alcohol that research has found may prevent cancer.

4. Celery

Celery is a popular vegetable found in a variety of cuisines from around the world. It can be eaten cooked or raw. In the United States, raw celery is served with spreads or dips as an appetizer. The wild celery plant had a coarse, earthy taste, and a distinctive smell.

With cultivation and blanching, the stalks lost their acidic qualities and assumed the mild, sweetish, aromatic taste particular to celery as a salad plant.

Celery contains many essential nutrients that our body needs to stay healthy. Celery is an excellent source of vitamin C which helps our body's immune system to fight off diseases. It also has a lot of potassium and folic acid both of which are important to keep your body functioning properly.

Celery is often called a "negative calorie food" but it certainly isn't lacking in nutrition. Celery is used in weight-loss diets, where it provides low-calorie dietary fiber bulk.

Celery, onions, and carrots are often used as a base for sauces and soups. Celery is a staple in many soups, such as chicken noodle soup, vegetable soup. It is also used in stews.

Celery seeds are used as flavoring or spice, either as whole seeds or ground and mixed with salt, as celery salt. Celery salt is also made from an extract of the roots, or using dried leaves. Celery salt is used as a seasoning, in cocktails, on the Chicago-style hot dog, and as seasoning.

Celery helps lower blood pressure by relaxing the muscles around the arteries and allowing vessels to dilate.

The calcium, magnesium, and potassium in celery also help regulate blood pressure.

Celery has been used as a diuretic for centuries. Its diuretic effect comes from its balance of potassium and sodium which helps to flush out excess fluid from the body.

Celery may also lower cholesterol by increasing bile acid secretion.

Celery is believed to have anti-inflammatory properties, which may help with ailments attributed to inflammation such as arthritis.

It is a great aid in weight loss because it is very low in calories and has a lot of filling fiber.

For medicinal use celery seeds and celery seed oil are also used.

Some people might get allergic to celery as celery is among a small group of foods (headed by peanuts) that appear to provoke the most severe allergic reactions; for people with celery allergy, exposure can cause potentially fatal.

5.   Cucumber

Cucumber is extremely beneficial to health especially during the summer as it mostly contains water and electrolytes. It also has many other important nutrients that are essential for human body. It is easy to grow and has many varieties, varying in size, shape, and color. Cucumber is best-harvested young, tender and just short of reaching maturity. At this stage they taste sweet, have crunchy texture, and unique flavor. Eat raw cucumber with skin. Cut cucumber for salads without peeling its skin. Cucumber peel is a good source of dietary fiber that helps reduce constipation.

Indian yellow curry-cucumber (*dosakayi*) is used widely in a variety of curry and stew preparations in south India with added buttermilk and yogurt.

Cucumber is known to heal many skin problems, under eye swellings and sunburn. It cools the eyes and the skin.

Cucumber is helpful in reducing cholesterol.

It prevents headaches, aids in weight loss, relieves joint pain, cures diabetes and controls blood pressure.

It contains no saturated fats or cholesterol. Cucumber offers some protection against colon cancers by eliminating toxic compounds from the gut.

The flesh of cucumber is rich in vitamins A, C, and folic acid while the hard skin of cucumber is rich in fiber and a range of minerals include magnesium, molybdenum, silica, and potassium.

In addition, cucumber has silica, a trace mineral contributing greatly at strengthening our connective tissues.

Cucumbers have a high amount of vitamin K. Vitamin-K has been found to have a potential role in bone strength by promoting osteotrophic (bone mass building) activity.

Cucumber also contains ascorbic and caffeic acids which prevent water loss.

Cucumber can be applied topically on burns and dermatitis.

Because cucumbers are 95% water they keep the body hydrated and help the body flush out toxins.

Cucumbers also help in diabetes, blood pressure, constipation, and bone health.

6.   Green Pepper

Green pepper is classified as a vegetable. There is a variety of green peppers. They come in many shapes and sizes. Some of them are sweet some are mild hot and some are very hot. Avoid very hot ones as they may be uncomfortable to your tongue and stomach. Bell peppers are sweet. They come in many colors and are delicious in salads, pasta and many other dishes. They add color to the meals.

The green pepper is very high in vitamin C. We get the benefit of this vitamin C if we eat fresh, raw peppers. They lose some of this vitamin C when cooked.

According to The World's Healthiest Foods, they may help prevent or reduce some of the symptoms of atherosclerosis and heart disease.

They can also help the nerve and blood vessel from damage seen in diabetes. They protect the eyes from the cloudy lenses of cataracts,. Peppers also help in releasing the joint pain and damage seen in osteoarthritis and rheumatoid arthritis. Eating green peppers help in the wheezing and airway tightening of asthma.

Peppers reportedly also have properties that regulate blood circulation, strengthen the heart, arteries and nerves, reduce the risk of flu, eliminate pain, relieve rheumatoid arthritis pain and reduce alcoholism, and boost your eyesight.

A 1-cup serving of green bell peppers contains 2.5 grams of fiber. If you take in enough fiber on a daily basis, your digestive system works more efficiently, which means you're less likely to get constipated or develop hemorrhoids. The fiber in peppers also helps prevent cancer of the colon.

Peppers are a low-calories food. Both green peppers and hot peppers have been shown to increase the body's heat production and oxygen consumption for about 20 minutes after eating. This causes your body to burn extra calories, which helps with weight loss.

Eat raw green bell peppers with low-fat ranch dressing or hummus for a nutritious and tasty side dish or snack.

Stir chopped green bell peppers into scrambled eggs or omelet.

Add finely chopped raw green bell pepper to tossed green salad or add to pasta salad.

Add it to different vegetable dishes for taste and flavor. Garnish meat and fish dishes with finely chopped green, red or yellow pepper.

Cook stuffed bell pepper. Use ground beef, lamb or chicken meat for stuffing. You can use mixed vegetable as well.

Slightly fried pepper can be added to potato, peas and cauliflower dishes.

7. Kale

Kale is called the "queen of greens". It is being recognized for its exceptional nutrient richness, health benefits, and delicious flavor. It is one of the more beautiful cruciferous vegetables, and is also one of the most nutritious.

One cup of kale has only 36 calories and zero grams of fat, which makes it a great diet aid. It promotes regular digestion, prevents constipation, lowers blood sugar and curbs overeating.

Kale is rich in carotenoids and flavonoids, two powerful antioxidants that protect our cells from free radicals that cause oxidative stress. Kale is also rich in the eye-health promoting lutein and zeaxanthin compounds.

Kale also provides a high dose of vitamin K that further aids to fight against excessive inflammatory-related problems, such as arthritis, autoimmune disorders, and asthma. Vitamin K is necessary for a protein that strengthens the composition of our bones. Vitamin K also prevents calcium build-up in our tissue that can lead to atherosclerosis, cardiovascular disease and stroke. Finally, vitamin K is essential to maintain the myelin sheath around our nerves, and therefore our nervous system as a whole.

One cup of kale is an effective antioxidant, boosts immunity, maintains healthy bones and teeth, prevents urinary stones, and is essential to our reproductive organs.

One cup of kale provides vitamin C, which is not only a powerful antioxidant, but also lowers blood pressure, ensures a healthy immune system, and fights against age-related ocular diseases, such as cataracts and macular degeneration.

Eat more kale if you have bowel movement problem.

A healthy diet of kale also provides glucosinolates, which have been shown to prevent colon, breast, bladder, prostate, ovarian cancers, as well as gastric cancer.

Kale is also known as "new Beef". Kale is low in calorie, high in fiber and has 0 fat. 1 cup of kale has only 36 calories, 5 grams of fiber and 0 grams of fat. It is also filled with so many nutrients, vitamins, folate and magnesium.

Kale is a beneficial, highly nutritious vegetable, prepared deliciously when steamed with diced onions, and garlic, a little bit of salt and pepper. Make juice of kale with cucumber, celery, green apples, lemon, and ginger, and is commonly known as the mean green juice. Have juice at least twice a week. It is good for sore throat and chills.

Lot of nutrients are lost when you steam or cook it. Eating it raw or juicing it is the best way. But some people do not like its taste and texture.

To prepare delicious crunchy kale just break it up into pieces place on cookie sheet drizzle olive oil, Put kale on a cookie sheet and sprinkle cheese of your choice on top of kale. Sprinkle a little salt and pepper if like and bake in oven on 375° for 10 to 15 minutes or until crispy. Enjoy crunchy kale chips.

Try kale banana smoothies, kale juice, steamed kale, sautéed kale. Try to buy organic kale because washing it isn't enough. The pesticides seep into the plant cells when they are grown in that stuff. You can't wash it off easily.

Avoid eating calcium-rich foods like dairy at the same time as kale to prevent any problems.

The benefits of kale just haven't gotten around to eating it more often. Have some sautéed kale with a nice glass of juice or water.

Eat kale for dinner in some form at least once a week. Eat kale for breakfast in a smoothie. Kale is really good for dieting.

8. Okra

Okra is a vegetable that is used in cuisines around the world. Okra is a non-starchy vegetable that can actually prevent your blood sugar levels from rising too high after your meals because of the special fiber it contains.

Okra is very low in calories and rich in fiber. It is a good source of vitamins A, C and K as well as folic acid and other important minerals. Okra contains a good source of iron and calcium. It also contains starch, fat, ash, thiamine and riboflavin.

- Okra also prevents constipation, gas and bloating in the abdomen.
- Some information shows that eating okra lowers the risk of cataracts.
- Okra is an excellent laxative and treats irritable bowels, heals ulcers and sooths the gastrointestinal track. The seeds of okra contain protein and oil and are good source of vegetable protein.
- The slime-like substance that forms on cooked okra actually is soluble fiber. The slime formed by soluble fiber from okra in your digestive tract can slow down the digestion of carbohydrates consumed at the same meal and delay the rise in your blood sugar levels. Okra can help prevent your blood sugar levels from going up, thus helping controlling your pre-diabetes or diabetes.
- The glycemix index (GI) is a measurement of how quickly carbohydrates in foods turn to sugar in your blood. Okra is classifies as having hypoglycemic properties. Regular consumption of okra can help keep our blood sugar levels balanced and aid in weight control. Okra has a GI below 20, which is considered a "low GI" food.

- Eating okra is much recommended for pregnant woman. It is rich in folic acid which is essential in the formation of the fetus during 4-12 weeks of gestation period in the mother's womb.
- Boil horizontally sliced okra till the brew become maximally slimy. Cool it and add a few drops of lemon and use this as the last rinse and see your hair will become bouncy and youthful.

9. Onions

I think onion is a widely used vegetable. It should be found in every kitchen. Cooking without onions especially meat dishes is like missing the most important ingredient. Onions have many health benefits and they are a very good source of vitamin C, B6, biotin, chromium, calcium and dietary fiber. In addition, they contain good amounts of folic acid and vitamin B1 and K.

They also contain flavonoids, which are pigments that give vegetables their color. These compounds act as antioxidants, have a direct antitumor effect and have immune-enhancing properties.

Onions contain a large amount of sulfur and are especially good for the liver. As a sulfur food, they mix best with proteins, as they stimulate the action of the amino acids to the brain and nervous system.

The onion is the richest dietary source of quercitin, a potent antioxidant flavonoid. Shallots, yellow and red onions also contain it but it is not in white onions.

Quercitin has been shown to thin the blood, lower cholesterol, raise good-type HDL cholesterol, ward off blood clots, fight asthma, chronic bronchitis, hay fever, diabetes, atherosclerosis and infections and is specifically linked to inhibiting human stomach cancer.

It's also an anti-inflammatory, antibiotic, antiviral, thought to have diverse anti-cancer powers. Quercitin is also a sedative. So far, there is no better food source of quercitin than onion skins.

You don't need to eat loads of onions to achieve these effects. In fact, studies show that you can eat just one medium onion, raw or cooked, a day. A 100 gram serving provides 44 calories.

Onions help to keep your blood free of clots.

Onions boost beneficial HDL cholesterol, and lower the triglycerides and lower total blood cholesterol. They are good for making the blood thin. They lower the blood pressure. Onions have been shown to have a significant blood sugar-lowering action. Onions have historically been used to treat asthma, too. Its action in asthma is due to its ability to inhibit the production of compounds that cause the bronchial muscle to spasm and to relax bronchial muscle.

Onions have potent antibacterial activity, destroying many disease-causing pathogens, including E. coli and salmonella. Lower total blood cholesterol.

In short these are the benefits of onions: improve immunity, regulate blood sugar, reduce inflammation, heal infection, antiseptic, antimicrobial, remedy for common cold, cough, fever and sore throat, increse sperm count, reduce pain and inflamation of joints.

Use of onions as well as garlic, leeks and shallots, seems a good idea due to their healing effects on the major degenerative diseases so common today, such as atherosclerosis, diabetes and cancer.

If unable to sleep cut an onion and massage the sole of your feet for few minutes. Its sedative effect will help you fall asleep.

Chop up a raw onion and cover it with honey and let it stand for four or five hours. It makes an excellent cough syrup and is wonderfully soothing for an inflamed throat.

Applying onion juice on the hair will eleminate lice.

Apply the mixture of onion juice with turmeric powder on face to remove dark pigments and patches. A drop of onion juice will soothe the ear ache.

People who use onions regularly will prevent tooth decay, and rubbing raw onion will temporarily reduce tooth pain. They may also help eleminate worms from the stomach of children.

If cuting onions makes your eyes tear or irritating put a amedium size nail in a bowl of water next to you. Hopefully your eyes will not tear or irritate.

10. Potatoes

Potato is a most widely used vegetable all over the world. Potato is an important global food source. After wheat and rice, potato is the third most important food crop, with a world-wide production of 309 million tons in 2007. While there are close to 4000 different varieties of potato, it has been bred into many standard or well-known varieties, such as russets, reds, whites, yellows (also called Yukons) and purples— based on common characteristics. Some potatoes are good for baking and some for boiling.

Potatoes aren't just about carbohydrates anymore. As a matter of fact there's growing evidence that potatoes may be among the most healthful vegetables around. Of course, it's best to bake a potato to get its full health benefits. A limited amount of potatoes should be eaten with each meal. If you are overweight or diabetic the intake of potatoes should be limited to one medium baked potato. At the same time it's important to check with your doctor, nutritionist and other health care professional about integrating potatoes into your daily diet and routine.

Potato is a member of species, such as tomato, eggplant, petunia, tobacco and pepper.

Potatoes provide the body with an essential source of fuel and energy, which you need even when dieting. Potatoes are a source of rich complex carbohydrate that is needed to our body for movement, thinking, digestion and cellular renewal.

It's nice to know that a new cooked potato has only 26 calories and is packe dwith nuttrients. Even then when people go on diet they cut down on potato after sugar.

Researchers at the Institute for Food Research in Norwich have found blood-pressure lowering molecules in potatoes called kukoamines. Traditional Chinese Medicine uses a plant, Lycium— which also contains kukoamines—as a tea to lower blood pressure. Good servings of potatoes a day would have some blood-pressure lowering activity as well.

The potato is best known for its carbohydrate content (26 grams in a medium potato). This carbohydrate comes from starch. It offers protection against colon cancer, improves glucose tolerance and insulin sensitivity, lowers plasma cholesterol and triglyceride concentrations, increases satiety, and possibly even reduces fat storage. (wikipedia)

After wheat and rice potatoes are third in number that are used for human consumption world wide. I had read a book titled "1000 ways of cooking potatoes" In every country there are different ways of cooking them. They are used in breakfast, in meals and in scacks. You will find some not very common recipes in the last chapter of this book.

11. Radish

- Radishes are related to mustard greens. Radishes come in variety of shapes and colors. They can be round or elongated, red, white, pink, purple and red-and-white. Some radishes have a very spicy flavor, while others are milder. Radishes are low-calorie vegetable. They contain essential nutrients and minerals that include potassium, manganese, magnesium, calcium, iron, phosphorous, sodium, copper and zinc.
- Radishes also have contents of vitamin C, B and K.

- Vitamin C works in the body to rebuild tissues, blood vessels and maintains bones and teeth. Vitamin K is beneficial for eyes.
- A ½-cup serving of radish slices contains only 19 calories.
- In Ayurvedic healing practices radishes are considered effective for toxin-purging effects.
- Even though they are considered gas producing radishes have a calming effect on the digestive system and can help relieve bloating and indigestion.
- They help in breaking down and eliminating toxins and cancer-causing free radicals in the body.
- Radishes can be eaten raw as they are cool and crunchy. They can be added to salads. Even radish leaves can be cooked as a vegetable with or without radishes. Radishes can be cooked mixed with other vegetables. They can be grilled, sautéed or cooked as curry.
- Eating radish regularly helps in urinary problems. For patients of jaundice boil radish in a quart of water for 15 minutes. Add some brown sugar to it and give it to patient every day.
- Eating radish and drinking butter milk with it also helps in treating jaundice.
- Radish takes time to digest but help other foods to digest fast. Eat raw brown sugar a little after eating radish to digest it. It will stop smelly burps also.
- For kidney stones consuming radish constantly helps break the stones and expel them easily.
- For liver health eat finely grated radish with salt.
- For bloody piles give the patient juice of radish to drink and radish leaves to eat, raw or cooked.
- For gums and teeth problems eat radish with ground black pepper.
- For asthma radish salt with honey helps if taken at least for 3 weeks.

12. Spinach

Spinach Is One of the Most Nutritious Foods Available. Spinach is a dark leafy green vegetable that provides a range of nutrients and essential vitamins. It can be eaten cooked or raw, or blended into smoothies to add a nutritious kick to health shakes.

Spinach is low in calories and high in nutritional value, making it a great addition to diets. Spinach is inexpensive and readily available both at local super markets and in grocery stores. It can also be grown relatively easily in a household garden.

Spinach is one of the most nutrient-dense foods in existence. Remember "Popeye the Sailor". He drew his energy from a can of spinach. It is an excellent source of more than 20 different measurable nutrients, including dietary fiber, calcium and protein. And yet, 1 cup has only 40 calories! Spinach is an excellent choice for nutrition without high calories.

One cup of the leafy green vegetable contains far more than your daily requirements of vitamin K and vitamin A, almost all the manganese and folate your body needs and nearly 40 percent of your magnesium requirement.

Spinach is packed with nutrients, including vitamins K, C, B1, B2, B6 and E, as well as carotenes, folic acid, manganese, magnesium and iron. Compared to most other greens, spinach contains twice as much iron per serving. Eating spinach increases strength.

Cancer-Fighting Antioxidants Abound in Fresh Spinach: Spinach contains more than a dozen individual flavonoid compounds, which work together as cancer-fighting antioxidants.

Scientific Research on Spinach

According to research compiled by Whole Foods, spinach is an excellent promoter of cardiovascular health. The antioxidant properties of spinach (water-soluble in the form of vitamin C and fat-soluble beta-carotene), work together to promote good cardiovascular health, by preventing the harmful oxidation of cholesterol. Oxidized cholesterol is a danger to the heart and arteries. Magnesium in spinach works toward healthy blood pressure levels. In fact, just a salad-size portion of spinach will work to lower high blood pressure within hours.

Eating Spinach Combats Ovarian, Prostate Cancers: The Journal of Nutrition reports that spinach contains a carotenoid that makes prostate cancers destroy themselves. This same carotenoid, after being changed by the intestines, prevents prostate cancer from reproducing itself.

Spinach also contains a strong antioxidant that prevents the formation of cancerous cells. Women who have a high intake of this flavonoid show a reduced risk of ovarian cancer. Spinach improves Brain Function, Protects against aging. This dark green leaf will protect your brain function from premature aging and slow old age's typical negative effects on your mental capabilities. Spinach prevents harmful effects of oxidation on your brain.

Those who eat vegetables in quantity, especially those of the leafy green variety, experience a decrease in brain function loss. Raw spinach retains more of its nutritional value, as the cooking process can leach some of the essential nutrients from the delicate leaves. Make a spinach salad by tossing spinach leaves with raw chopped vegetables and nuts. Raw spinach is a great ingredient to add to health shakes to quickly and easily increase the nutritional value. Add raw spinach leaves to sandwiches in place of lettuce, which contains far fewer nutrients, or simply munch on spinach leaves as a snack throughout your day.

One cup of spinach has nearly 20% of the FDA of dietary fiber, which aids in digestion, prevents constipation, maintains low blood sugar, and curbs overeating.

Neoxanthin and violaxanthin are two anti-inflammatory epoxyxanthophylls that play an important role in regulation of inflammation and are present in unusual amounts in spinach.

The vitamin C, vitamin E, beta-carotene, manganese, zinc and selenium present in spinach all serve as powerful antioxidants that combat the onset of osteoporosis, atherosclerosis and high blood pressure. One cup of spinach contains over 337% of the FDA of vitamin A that not only protects and strengthens "entry points" into the human body, such as mucous membranes, respiratory, urinary and intestinal tracts, but is also a key component of lymphocytes (or white blood cells) that fight infection.

The high amount of vitamin A in spinach also promotes healthy skin by allowing for proper moisture retention in the epidermis, thus fighting psoriasis, acne and even wrinkles.

Vitamin K is a crucial component of the process called carboxylation, which produces the matrix Gla protein that directly prevents calcium from forming in tissue. Eating one cup of spinach contributes to this process that fights atherosclerosis, cardiovascular disease and stroke.

The abundance of vitamin K in spinach contributes greatly to a healthy nervous system and brain function by providing an essential part for the synthesis of sphingolipids, the crucial fat that makes up the Myelin sheath around our nerves.

Flavonoids a phytonutrient with anti-cancer properties abundant in spinach—have been shown to slow down cell division in human stomach and skin cancer cells. Furthermore, spinach has shown significant protection against the occurrence of aggressive prostate cancer.

Before cooking with fresh spinach, make sure to wash it thoroughly, as loose bunches and packaged leaves tend to hold dirt. Cook it using any kind of recipes it is good for your health.

13. Sweet Potatoes

Sweet Potatoes are highly nutritious. Sweet potatoes contain vitamin A, vitamin C, manganese, fiber, B vitamins, potassium and even iron. In fact, Whole Foods considers sweet potatoes one of the healthiest vegetables we eat.

Diabetics can eat sweet potatoes without worry as these tubers have a low glycemic index.

Vitamins A and C are also anti-inflammatory, making sweet potatoes an excellent food for those suffering from either form of arthritis or asthma.

If you suffer from kidney or gallbladder ailments, talk with your doctor or health care professional about a recommended intake of sweet potatoes.

Bake them, boil them or microwave them. They taste sweet and good. Bake sweet potato pies.

Make pudding just the way you make rice pudding. It tastes delicious.

You may boil or micro wave sweet potatoes. Peel and slice them. Serve them hot.

14. Tomato

A Tomato is red and usually has four chambers, just like our heart. But tomatoes come in many colors, and have many varieties: beef tomatoes, plum tomatoes, cherry tomatoes. Eat raw or cooked they are full of nutrients and very healthy vegetable. They are easy to grow.

Tomatoes are also a great source of lycopene, a plant chemical that reduces the risk of heart disease and several cancers.

The Women's Health Study an American research program which tracks the health of 40,000 women found women with the highest blood levels of lycopene had 30 per cent less heart disease than women who had very little lycopene. One Canadian study, published in the journal Experimental Biology and Medicine, said there was convincing evidence that lycopene prevented coronary heart disease.

Daily consumption of tomato provides a good boost to health. Use of tomato is good for heart disease, hypertension, cardiovascular disease, urinary infection, and asthma and chronic lung disease. Tomato is helpful in atherosclerosis and diabetes. Use of tomato is good for vision, strong and shiny hair, and healthy skin. It is helpful in reducing inflammation.

Cooking process doesn't destroy important nutrients of tomato.

Spaghetti sauce is made from cooked tomatoes and provides key nutrients.

Eat cooked tomatoes with a small amount of food that contains fat, such as olive oil or cheese.

Use cooked tomatoes in pasta recipes or add them to rice to make a nutritious Spanish rice side dish.

Add cooked tomatoes to soup, chili and casseroles.

Add sliced tomatoes, tomato paste or tomato sauce when cooking meat curries.

Bake tomatoes.

Grill them. Or eat them raw.

Use raw tomatoes in salads.

If you grow tomatoes in your backyard you may freeze extra ones for the winter use.

Chapter 4

NUTS AND SEEDS

Nuts and seeds are popular foods in many diets. They are often eaten as snacks. But in most vegetarian dishes they are main element. These nuts and seeds are so nutrient-dense that they are called powerhouses of protein, fiber, healthy fats, enzymes and a number of vitamins and minerals. All nuts help in lowering LDL the bad cholesterol. They keep blood pressure in check.

People enjoy eating whole nuts and seeds or they are used in many recipes of meat and rice. Nut creams and nut milks are also used to make sauces or in smoothies.

We should store all seeds and nuts in a cool and dry place, and in an airtight container. Since nuts and seeds have a high unsaturated fat content, they may lose their taste or smell if not handled properly. Nuts in the shell will keep longer than shelled nuts. But it is convenient to use the shelled ones.

Add some bay leaves and a cinnamon stick to the storage containers of the nuts and seeds and they will stay fresh. Since they retain the highest level of enzymes and other nutritional value that way it is best to eat them raw. They are also easy to digest than roasted nuts due to the enzymatic activity of raw foods.

Seeds should be bought whole and if need be ground fresh.

1. Almonds

Almonds are chock full of vitamins. There's vitamin E to bolster the immune system, vitamin E is a very important antioxidant, plus a range of B vitamins, which may make the body more resilient during bouts of stress such as depression. Key to health is eating a handful of almonds.

They are dense in vitamins and minerals that help keep your body healthy. Almonds also provide a hefty dose of protein and fiber, and contain the essential fatty acids omega-3 and omega-6. They also contain zinc, calcium, iron, phosphorus, potassium, and magnesium. Fat in almonds is mono-saturated fat, which is great for heart (also found in olive oil and salmon. This means it helps neutralize free radicals, which if unchecked, can result in disease and illness. Almonds can also help you lose weight. They contain fiber, protein, and the good type of fat. They help keep you full, making them an ideal healthy snack. If you fill up on almonds, you won't need to grab those potato chips or cookies.

Most importantly, almonds are very beneficial for heart health. They also keep your brain cells healthy. They contain low levels of saturated fat and have no cholesterol. According to the U.S. Food and Drug Administration eating almonds will not only help you avoid food that is unhealthy, but almonds themselves can actually help you maintain your health.

According to Almond Board of California the leading cause of death in men and women in the United States is heart disease. The Almond Board of California actually recommends eating 23 almonds a day for maximum health benefits. They are good for eyes, sugar control and also for memory.

Almonds are low on the gylcemic index, which means they do not cause a large increase in blood glucose levels. It has been found that almonds help decrease rises in blood sugar after meals. This can help prevent the development of diabetes.

Some Home Remedies

- Soak 7 almonds overnight. Peel the skin in the morning. Eat them chewing well. Good for headache and eyes.
- You may also add a ½ cup of milk and ½ spoon of honey and blend the ingredients in a blender. Pour it in a glass, add 2 ice cubes and drink a soothing cold drink. You may double the quantity and save half of it for the next morning. Drink it at least one hour before taking breakfast. This drink will give you energy, relieve headache and make you feel fresh for the day.
- Almond oil is also available. It has the ability to soften and condition the skin. It also helps lighten dark complexion. It can be used as a moisturizer.
- Almond oil is also very good for hair. Its use will stop your hair from falling. You need to give your scalp massage every day with almond oil. Soon the hair will stop falling and your hair will become healthier and longer.

- Almond oil can be used for cooking as well. But it can be used only in very small amount and only in some recipes. It is thick and very concentrated.

2. Basil Seeds

Basil leaves have many healing qualities. In India the Basil plant is revered for its benefits and is frequently used for minor ailments in children and also in adults. But basil seeds are also very beneficial for certain ailments and make a good remedy without any side effects.

Basil seeds sharpen memory. Use them as a nerve tonic. They are helpful in removing phlegm from your bronchial tubes. Repeat up to once an hour. The seeds can be used to rid the body of excess mucus.

The basil seed is called "tukmaria" for its health benefit rather than the whole plant. The tukmaria seed is black in color and slightly smaller than a grain of rice. It's available in small packs of 100grams in Asians market and cost approximately $2.90 per pack.

Basil seed or tukmaria is used for the treatment for constipation, indigestion and heartburn. Soak one teaspoon full of seeds in water overnight. Add some sugar or honey to taste and give a glass of tukmaria drink for indigestion or bloating resulting from bad eating. It can be taken anytime but the best is at night before going to bed. During the night while sleeping, it works as a cleanser to remove the toxin from the bowels and the next morning everything is flushed, and you are back to normal.

Basil drink is very simple to prepare. Just put a small amount (1-2 teaspoonful) of the basil seed soaked in water, after 30 minutes a jelly is formed around each seed. Simply add sugar to it and drink. Basil seed is tasteless. Milk or any other flavor may be added to the drink. Basil seed drink is very popular in Asian countries especially during summer time.

Adding falooda to basil drink is also very popular. Falooda is a cold and sweet beverage. It contains many ingredients and is a very popular drink in South Asia. Traditionally it is made by mixing rose or almond syrup with vermicelli, psyllium (ispaghol) or basil seeds. Jelly pieces and tapioca pearls along with either milk, water or ice cream are added to the drink. The vermicelli used are often made from arrowroot rather than wheat. The rose syrup may be substituted with another flavoured base to produce kesar (saffron), mango, chocolate or fig flavor.

Nowadays falooda is a popular summer drink throughout Pakistan, India, Bangladesh, Sri Lanka, Myanmar, and the Middle East and is readily available in restaurants and beach stalls.

It is a very thirst quenching and satisfying drink.

Basil seeds benefit people with constipation or diarrhea. Researchers believe that basil seeds may prevent sugar absorption by providing dietary fiber and relieve constipation by acting as a bulk-forming laxative.

Another benefit of basil seeds is that they also provide relief from influenza, fever and cold. Since it has antispasmodic effects, it can help treat whooping cough. In fact, tulsi (basil) is the main ingredient in many expectorants and cough syrups.

Consumption of basil seeds has an uplifting effect on your mood and thus is beneficial for relieving mental fatigue, nervous tension, melancholy, depression and migraine. Due to its calming effect, it is commonly used for aromatherapy purposes, giving you clarity and mental strength.

Oil is also extracted from basil seeds. It helps in treating infections such as wounds, cuts, bladder infections, skin infections etc. There is no evidence whatsoever that basil seeds have undesirable side effects. However, you should consult your doctor before you consume them, especially if you are on medication.

3.   Cashews

Cashews are very popular in South Asia. They are a primary ingredient in many Asian dishes and are packed with vitamins and minerals.

You can snack on these seeds raw, roasted, or as a cashew nut butter spread. You can find them chocolate coated, candied or coated with spices. Either way they make a good snack. Roasted cashews are most popular. Roasted cashews are a delicious and healthy snack. You can save money by buying raw nuts and roasting them yourself or have them honey coated. "Kaju Berfi" is a delicious sweet treat that you can buy from any Indian stores.

Sometimes cashew nuts are called "nature's vitamin pill," They were ranked #1 among nut crops in the world with 4.1 billion pounds produced in 2002. In one ounce of cashews 5 grams of protein is found along with high levels of the essential minerals iron, magnesium, phosphorus, zinc, copper and manganese, which are utilized in holistic health solutions and healthy diets.

With no cholesterol cashew nuts are healthy food for heart patients. They also support healthy levels of HDL the good cholesterol. Raw cashews may especially help lower the risk of developing Type 2 Diabetes. It is the most commonly diagnosed form of diabetes in America today.

Magnesium deficiencies can lead to an increase in blood pressure, muscle cramps and muscle spasms. These spasms include spasms of the heart and lungs. A 1/4 cup serving of cashews contains 23 percent of the recommended daily value of magnesium.

Magnesium with calcium helps support healthy muscles and bones in the human body. It also helps promote normal sleep patterns in menopausal women. Cashew's has high copper content is vital in energy production, greater flexibility in blood vessels, bones and joints.

Cashew nut helps the body utilize iron, eliminate free radicals, develop bone and connective tissue, and produce the skin and hair pigment melanin.

4. Fennel Seeds

Fennel seeds are the edible seeds of the fennel plant. They taste similar to licorice, are often used as a culinary spice, and can also be eaten or chewed raw. Chewing fennel seeds after meals is a great way to aid in digestion. In Indian sub-continent it is very customary to chew fennel seeds after the meal. You may chew ¼ spoon of fennel seed after meals to cleanse your mouth of bad breath and make it smelling fresh. Sometimes an almond and or a cardamom may be added for fresh breath.

Fennel seeds are high in fiber. Fiber helps balance the metabolism, aids in digestion and cleanses the colon. Fennel seeds can help prevent constipation, cleanse the body's digestive system, and aid the stomach in the formation of bile and other digestive juices.

Fennel seed water (boiled, strained and cooled) helps babies to burp, and reduces bloating and gas problem. Add a little bit of sugar or honey if the baby is one or older. Gripe Water is a good remedy for babies to help them to burp, and reduces bloating and gas problem. It is a European product, but it can be found in Indo-Pakistani stores.

Iron is essential for muscle function, brain function and the formation of hemoglobin. Irion deficiency can lead to severe body fatigue and conditions such as anemia. Fennel seeds are a good source of iron. It is essential for muscle function, brain function and the formation of hemoglobin. Iron deficiency can lead to severe body fatigue and conditions such as anemia. Chewing fennel seeds after meals can help in many of these conditions.

Fennel seeds also provide the required quantity of calcium which is essential in maintaining healthy teeth and bones and may also provide cardiovascular support.

The antioxidants in fennel seeds have anti-inflammatory properties. They may be an effective treatment for arthritis and Crohn's disease; however more research is still needed to confirm these reports.

The antioxidants in fennel seeds can help reduce cancer risk associated with free radical damage to cells and DNA. They also work alongside fiber to cleanse the colon and protect from colorectal cancer.

Fennel seeds are high in the antioxidant group known as flavonoids. Studies have found that flavonoids are effective combatants of free radical damage to cells in the body, a known cause of many different types of cancer.

Flavonoids can also help reduce oxidative stress to the cardiovascular system and protect from neurological disease.

Some reports claim that chewing fennel seed may help to reduce the symptoms of asthma, clear sinuses, and stabilize breathing. More research is needed to confirm the connection between fennel and healthy breathing.

There are some remedies to protect and to increase your eyesight by using fennel seeds:

- Eat 1 spoon of fennel seeds and 7 almonds every night. Constant use for at least 6 months will improve your eyesight.
- Use the blender pulsing it to get the outer layer of fennel seeds off. Take a spoon of these fennel seeds with milk at night. Continue using it. Your eyesight will not decrease.
- Fennel seeds and almond of same weight and 50% sugar candy or brown sugar grind them and make them into a powder. Take a spoon of this powder with warm milk. Do not drink water after that. See the difference in your eyesight in 40 days. My niece had used it and in six month she got rid of her glasses. Eyesight had improved to normal.

5. Flax Seeds

Some call it one of the most powerful plant foods on the planet. There's some evidence it may help reduce your risk of heart disease, cancer, stroke, and diabetes. These days all kind of foods and snacks have flaxseed in them from crackers to frozen waffles to many kinds of cereals. The Flax Council estimates close to 300 new flax-based products were launched in the U.S. and Canada in 2010 alone.

Although flaxseed contains all sorts of healthy components, but primarily most important healthy components are Omega-3 essential fatty acids, Lignans, and fiber.

One tablespoon of ground flaxseed contains 2 grams of polyunsaturated fatty acids (includes the omega 3s) and 2 grams of dietary fiber and 37 calories. Flaxseeds also have antioxidant properties, which may contribute to protection against cancer and heart disease.

Lignans have both plant estrogen and antioxidant qualities. Flaxseed contains 75 to 800 times more lignans than other plant foods. The lignans in flaxseed may provide some protection against cancers.

Flaxseed contains both the soluble and insoluble fiber.

An unbalanced diet can cause up to 15 pounds of waste to build up in your colon. The best way to get rid of that waste from your colon is to maintain high-fiber diet. Adding flex seeds in your diet is an excellent way to start your colon cleansing.

Flax seeds are also good for digestion and detoxifying cells.

Flax seed are anti-inflammatory and help gastrointestinal system.

They are also helpful in building up immune system.

Use flax seeds to help nervous system and to reduce stress.

Women who are suffering from hot flashes should use flex seeds to reduce them.

You may buy seeds or powder of flex seeds. Flex seeds can be added to your cereal in the morning, on your salads at meal time. You may take a spoon of flex seed powder at night time.

Adding a tablespoon of ground flaxseed to your hot or cold breakfast cereal will be easy and helpful for digestion.

You can also mix a tablespoon of ground flaxseed in plain or fruity yogurt.

Easy way to make a sandwich is to add a teaspoon of ground flaxseed to mayonnaise or mustard. Spread it on the slice of bread and enjoy it.

If you bake cup cakes, muffins, breads and other goods you may mix a spoon of powdered flex seeds in the batter before you bake them.

Most nutrition experts recommend ground flex seeds. They are better than whole flaxseed because the ground form is easier for your body to digest. Whole flaxseed may pass through your intestine undigested, which means you won't get all the benefits.

6. Peanuts

Peanut are lso known as ground nuts. They belong to beans and peas family. Peanuts are the best sources of protein. Peanuts are found in a wide variety of products. You can eat peanut salted, dry roasted, boiled and even raw. Peanut brittle, peanut butter and candy bars are all made with peanuts of course. In mixed nuts peanuts have a major portion. Some people like to boil raw peanuts. They taste as good as any way you eat them and maintain their health benefits.

Everyone likes peanuts. But some people and children are allergic to peanuts and many other nuts. They must be very careful about reading the ingredients in any product they buy. Sometimes the allergic reactions are very severe and need doctor's care and even hospitalization in some cases.

Peanuts help promote fertility (Folate). A ¼ cup of peanuts can supply the body with 35% of manganese, a mineral which helps metabolize the fat and carbohydrate, and help regulate blood sugar and absorb calcium.

Peanuts can help prevent gallstones. Twenty years of studies have shown that eating 1 ounce of nuts, peanuts or peanut butter a week lowers the risk of developing gallstones by 25%.

Peanuts are good sources of tryptophan, an essential amino acid which is important for the production of serotonin, one of the key brain chemicals involved in mood regulation.

People feeling depressed should eat peanuts to reduce their stress level. Vitamin B3 or niacin content found in peanuts have given them a name of "brain food".

The same nutrient which gives peanuts their memory enhancing power also helps lower and control cholesterol levels. Peanuts aid in reducing bad cholesterol and increase good cholesterol levels.

Regular nuts consumption is linked to reduced risk of heart disease. Peanuts are rich in heart-friendly monounsaturated fats and antioxidants such as oleic acid. Eating peanuts and other nuts at least four times a week will reduce the risk of cardiovascular and coronary heart disease.

Eating nuts regularly is associated with a lowered risk of weight gain.

7. Pistachios

Pistachios are small and green nuts. They are bought in shells or without them. As they say good things come in small package, it is very true for the nutrition benefits of pistachios. Another good thing is that it is a snack that does much more than curb your appetite. These nuts improve cardiovascular health and maintain vision. Pistachios contain a variety of nutrients. Some of those nutrients and their associated benefits are not always found in other nuts.

You may eat a handful of pistachios as a snack and get benefited by these healthy rewards.

Pistachios, as well as other nuts and seeds, are a great source of omega-3 fatty acids. Eating pistachios, walnuts, or almonds every day may help lower your cholesterol, reduce inflammation in the arteries of the heart, lower the risk of diabetes, and protect you against stress.

Pistachios also contain fiber which is beneficial for gastrointestinal health.

Pistachios are high in heart healthy monounsaturated fatty acids. Some studies have shown a decrease in LDL or bad cholesterol, and others have also shown an increase in HDL or good cholesterol. One study by Penn State University evaluated the influence of pistachio intake on blood pressure in response to stress.

Pistachios contain two unique carotenoids not often found in other nuts. The lutein and zeaxanthin act as protective antioxidants. Lutein and zeaxanthin have been associated with eye health and reduction of the risk for developing age-related macular degeneration which is the leading cause of blindness in the United States.

Pistachios are an excellent source of copper, manganese and Vitamin B6, as well as a good source of a variety of other B vitamins.

Copper is important as it helps in the formation of connective tissue.

Manganese is important for tissue development, growth, reproduction and the metabolism of fat and carbohydrates.

Vitamin B6 is important in the development of antibodies within the immune system.

Vitamin B6 assists with healthy nerve function and the production of red blood cells.

It is important to watch portion sizes. Though nutritious, they are also high in calorie which can ruin weight loss efforts. Pistachios are not lower calorie nuts. A serving of pistachios is about 50 nuts, providing 170 calories. Pistachios in the shell are heavily salted. Avoid them as excess sodium does raise blood pressure in some people.

You can store pistachios in an airtight container for up to three months in the fridge or freeze them for six months. If you want to store them for a longer period of time put a few bay leaves and a cinnamon stick in the container. They will stay fresh and would not stale.

Pistachios are used in ice creams, in different drinks, in many Asian and Middle Eastern sweets, in yogurts. You can use them in baking goods at home to reap the health benefits of these nuts, or just munch on them.

8.   Pumpkin Seeds

Pumpkin seeds have long been valued as a source of the mineral zinc, and the World Health Organization recommends their consumption as a good way of obtaining this nutrient.

Zinc is especially concentrated in this endosperm envelope, the inner line in the shell. It would be good to eat the whole seed along with the shell.

Whole roasted, unshelled pumpkin seeds contain about 10 milligrams of zinc per 3.5 ounces, and shelled roasted pumpkin seeds contain about 7-8 milligrams. Eating with shells will increase your zinc intake.

Pumpkin seeds are a very good source of the minerals phosphorus, magnesium, and manganese, and a good source of the minerals zinc, iron, and copper.

Pumpkin seed extracts, and pumpkin seed oil have long been valued for their anti-microbial benefits, including their anti-fungal and anti-viral properties.

The oil in pumpkin seeds alleviates difficult urination that happens with an enlarged prostate.

In many cultures pumpkin seeds are used as a natural treatment for tapeworms and other parasites. Pumpkin seeds also help prevent kidney stone formation.

Pumpkin seeds are relatively large in size and are easy to crack open to eat. In Mexican culture these seeds are used in many food recipes. You may roast pumpkin seeds or spice them. If you prefer more savory snacks use garlic, onion and chili powders, or spicy seasonings and roast them. You may also use them as a topping on salads and cooked vegetables. Add to your favorite hot and cold cereals, granola or trail mix. For added protein, crush or grind the seeds and add to your meat or veggie burgers.

9. Sunflower Seeds

Sunflower seeds have been commonly included in various kinds of recipes and snacks due to the several health benefits stored in them. These seeds are a power house of unsaturated fats, 90% of these seeds comprise unsaturated fat. These seeds are also stuffed with vitamins, minerals, poly and monounsaturated fats, proteins and fibers.

Eat them raw or roasted they are a healthy snack. Sunflower seeds have vitamin E. It helps in reducing the ill effect of free radicals in the body. They help protecting the cell membranes and brain cells.

Asthma, colon cancer, cardiovascular diseases, and Rheumatoid Arthritis (RA), can also be treated by including these seeds in the diet. Vitamin E contents in sunflower seeds can also help improving blood clotting and wound healing.

These seeds add protein in the diet and become helpful in the maintenance, growth and repair of tissues.

These seeds are also rich in magnesium, which takes care of spasms, lowers the risk of hypertension, asthma attacks and migraines.

Sunflower seeds are a rich source of linolenic acid, which helps in removing the blockage in the blood capillaries and improvises circulation.

10. Walnuts

Walnuts are the only nuts that are significantly high in Omega 3s (alpha lenolenic acid also known as ALA).

Walnuts are also a source of protein, antioxidants, fiber, magnesium and phosphorus. Walnuts are packed with polyunsaturated fats and have been shown in clinical trials to help decrease your risk of heart disease by lowering cholesterol.

Walnuts contain magnesium (45 mg per ounce) a good source of energy. Eating about 14-21 halves of walnuts every day is an easy way to boost your daily nutrition. They are not only good for heart health but also for bone health and in managing type 2 diabetes.

If a child is in the habit of bed-wetting give him 4 halves of walnuts and 20 raisins to eat before he goes to bed for two weeks. Hopefully he will quit the habit.

Eating roasted walnuts in winter time will help the seasonal cold.

A walnut a day may keep bad cholesterol away, according to a 2010 study in the Archives of Internal Medicine that found a 7.4 percent reduction in "bad" LDL cholesterol and an 8.3 percent reduction in the ratio of LDL to HDL.(reported WebMD) What's more, triglyceride concentrations declined by more than 10 percent.

If you eat walnuts with figs it is helpful in intoxicating the body.

Eat 8 halves of walnuts, 4 almonds and 10 large raisins in the morning and drink cold milk with it. It will give you energy and will be especially good in winter time.

Grind walnuts and mix them with vinegar to prepare a mask. Apply on face and wash it as soon as it dries up. This mask will make you skin soft and glowing.

Walnut is diuretic; it will help those who have difficulty in urinating with strong flow.

If your calorie needs are less than 2000 calories a day, you probably want to stick to about 14 halves a day.

You may use chopped walnuts in your breakfast cereal. Use walnuts as topping on your ice cream.

Make a creamy dip with Greek yogurt and walnuts. Add finely chopped parsley/ cilantro and one clove of finely crushed garlic.

Use them in smoothes. Add walnuts to yogurt.

Make walnut butter by blending them in food processor until they are smooth. Add some honey and a little bit of cinnamon. Walnut butter is ready just like peanut butter.

Walnuts take time to digest. Do not eat too many walnuts. Just limit it to 14 to 21 walnut halves a day. Eating too many walnuts may cause headache and sometimes soar mouth.

Chapter 5

SPICES AND HERBS

People had been using herbs and spices from time unknown for many purposes. These herbs and spices were being used in foods for aroma flavor of them. Some spices were burned in the house to make it smell good or to get rid of bad smell. They were being used for treatment of some common ailments. Some of these herbs and spices are still being used for their healing properties and they work. Before going to a physician use them. Save time and money. Worry not for any side effects as they are nature's medicines. If they do not help they will not harm. If some ailment still persists then it is time for you to go and see a doctor.

1. Basil Leaves

Basil is an aromatic herb of the mint family. Another variety of it is called sweet basil. Fresh or dried leaves are used for seasoning of many dishes. In Indian sub-continent it is used for many common ailments. It is called "Tulsi" the healing herb. Leaves can strengthen the stomach and induce perfuse sweating. The herb is useful in the cure of respiratory disease, according to recent studies. A mixture of the herb, with ginger and honey is a remedy for asthma, cough, cold, influenza and bronchitis. Simply boil it in a glass of water and consume it just like tea.

Make tea with basil leaves and drink it when your body is very tired. It will relax you.

If having earache take out the juice of some basil leaves and put couple of drops in the ear. It will help relieve the pain.

If you keep the tulsi plant in the house malaria spreading mosquitoes will not come. Apply juice of tulsi leaves on face and arms and any exposed areas of your body the mosquitoes will not bite you.

Rub dry leaves on the face to give it a fresh look.

Rubbing the basil leaves on ringworm might help cure it.

For black spots on the face grind some basil leaves into a paste add some lemon juice and apply on the face. It will clean the black spots.

For cold and cough among children grind new baby leaves of tulsi (basil) add some honey and give ½ a spoon before bedtime. It will give quick relief.

Basil is an important ingredient in cough syrups and expectorants. It can also relieve mucus in asthma and bronchitis. Chewing on basil leaves can relieve colds and flu symptoms.

Water boiled with basil leaves can be taken as a tonic or used as a gargle when you have a sore throat.

Basil leaves are used for bringing down the temperature especially when the fever is related to malaria and other infectious, eruptive fevers common to tropical areas. Boiling leaves with some cardamom in about two quarts of water, then mixed with sugar and milk, brings down temperature. An extract of basil leaves in fresh water should be given every 2 to 3 hours; between doses you can give sips of cold water. This method is especially effective for reducing fevers in children.

Boiling the leaves, cloves, and sea salt in some water will give rapid relief of influenza. These combinations should be boiled in about two quarts of water until only half the water remains before they are taken.

Basil can be used to strengthen your kidneys. It is a long term remedy but it will help. Kidney will expel them through the urinary tract if basil leaves' juice is mixed with honey and taken daily.

Basil can also reduce your cholesterol. It will purify the blood and help prevent many other common ailments.

Juice of basil leaves in pediatric complaints like colds, coughs, fever, diarrhea, and vomiting has been known to respond well. Basil leaves can be used as an anti-stress agent. Chew 12 basil leaves twice a day to prevent stress. Chewing a few leaves twice daily can cure infections and ulcerations of the mouth.

Basil can be used preventatively and as a curative. A teaspoonful of the basil leaf juice taken every few hours is preventative. Rubbing the bites of insects and leeches with basil juice to relieve the itching and swelling is curative. Also a paste of the root is effective for treating the bites.

Basil juice applied directly to the affected area is good for ringworm and other common skin ailments.

People in Asian cultures dry basil leaves in the sun and grind into powder for a tooth cleansing powder and by mixing it with mustard oil to make herbal toothpaste. Both of these methods will kill bad breath and would be therapeutic to massage the gums, treat pyorrhea, and other dental hygiene.

Basil is a good headache remedy. Boil leaves in half a quart of water, cooking until half the liquid remains. Take a couple of teaspoons an hour with water to relieve your pain and swelling. You can also make a paste of basil leaves pounded with sandalwood to apply to your forehead to relieve headache and provide coolness in general.

Basil juice is good for night-blindness and sore eyes. Two drops of black basil juice in each eye at bedtimes each day is soothing.

At the end I should say that basil is the herb that should be in every household and be used to prevent certain conditions and to cure many ailments. This is the best home remedy that you may grow in your back yard or even indoors in a pot.

2. Cardamom

Cardamom is commonly known in Indian sub-continent as "choti elaichi". Cardamom's scientific name is Elletaria cardamomum. Cardamom is popularly used as a herbal spice.

It is added in dishes to provide a strong and pleasant aroma and flavor. It is considered to be a very useful and effective medicine as well.

Cardamom is effective in improving digestion. It helps stomach cramps and is good stimulant and beneficial for those suffering from indigestion and gas.

Cardamom has detoxifying properties. It helps cleansing the body. It is basically a warm spice and known to have originated from India. It improves blood circulation to the lungs and can be helpful in preventing spasms or convulsions. Cardamom therefore is beneficial for those suffering from asthma or bronchitis, but is should be taken in small quantity. The quantity of cardamom which needs to be consumed depends on the physiology of a person and the disease which is to be treated or cured from.

Cardamom enhances appetite and provides relief from acidity in the stomach. It is used in the cure of halitosis. It is beneficial for those suffering from various kinds of respiratory allergies.

For sore throat make tea with cardamom, add some honey and drink sipping it as hot as you can tolerate. Best thing is make green tea added with couple of "choti ilaichis." Elaichi tea is also very aromatic and refreshing.

If you are suffering from nausea try to chew a few cardamom seeds. Some practitioners advise using cardamom for treating infection of the urinary tract.

For treating mouth ulcers cardamom can be used along with any other medicine. It is known to be a good cure for weakness in general. Just chew "ilaichi" seeds as mouth freshner after meals. Add ilaichi to your rice dishes for its aroma and flavor. Use ground ilaichi to garnish sweet dishes for good taste. Just sprinkle a pinch or two on top. For tea lovers it would be good experience to try Tetley's ilaichi Tea bags.

3.   Cinnamon

Cinnamon is a spice obtained from the inner bark of several trees from the genus *Cinnamomum* that is used in both sweet and savory foods. Cinnamon has long been a popular spice in baking and cooking. Research has found that it is not only delicious but it's healthy too. Just make sure that you're not buying cassia, which is often sold as cinnamon in stores.

Cinnamon should be included in our diet every day. For health benefits several studies have shown that just 1/2 teaspoon of cinnamon per day can lower LDL cholesterol. If you have type 2 diabetes cinnamon may have a regulatory effect on blood sugar.

Cinnamon has shown an amazing ability to stop yeast infections that were known to be medication-resistant.

As a home remedy take half a teaspoon of cinnamon powder combined with one tablespoon of honey every morning before breakfast for relief in arthritis pain. After one or two week you will see significant relief in pain and with its continuous use you might be able to walk without pain within a month or so.

If you have regular use of a teaspoon of cinnamon it will help lower your LDL cholesterol, and will also help preventing blood clotting. These three reasons are enough for any one suffering from these ailments (arthritis, bad cholesterol LDL and blood clotting) to use cinnamon in your daily diet.

In one study published by researchers at the U.S. Department of Agriculture in Maryland, it was said that cinnamon reduced the proliferation of leukemia and lymphoma cancer cells.

Cinnamon is used widely in so many sweet dishes and desserts. Don't you love cinnabuns?

It is sprinkled on rice pudding.

In many Indo-Pakistani sweet dishes, rice dishes and even some meat dishes cinnamon is used for its' strong flavor and of course for its health benefits.

4. Cloves

Cloves are nature's top anti-oxidant food. They are native to the Spice Islands of Indonesia. They have been consumed in Asia for more than 2,000 years. Owing to their sweet and fragrant taste, Chinese courtiers dating back to 200 BC would keep them in their mouths in order to freshen up their breath when addressing the emperor so as not offend him with their bad breaths. Arab traders brought cloves to Europe around the 4th century.

Cloves can be bought easily in any supermarket and Asian stores throughout the year. They have a uniquely warm, sweet, spicy and aromatic taste. People have been using them in ginger bread and pumpkin pies for centuries. They make a wonderful addition to split pea and bean soups, baked beans and chili. "Biryani" a famous Asian dish has flavor of cloves in it. A sweet rice dish called "Zarda" cloves are used in it. In some other sweet dishes cloves are used for their aroma and flavor.

For toothache use clove oil. Its anesthetic properties soothe pain. Chew a clove a little bit and put it on the aching tooth. It will help take away inflammation.

Just keep one clove in your mouth to take away the bad breath.

Although most spices are excellent sources of antioxidants, cloves rank as the richest source of them all. For centuries people had known the health benefits of cloves. Cloves have antiseptic and germicidal properties that help fight infections, relieve digestive problems and arthritis pain.

Eugenol, the primary component of clove's volatile oils, functions as an anti-inflammatory substance. Clove also contains a variety of flavonoids, including kaempferol and rhamnetin, which also contribute to clove's anti-inflammatory (and antioxidant) properties.

Clove is an excellent source of manganese, a very good source of omega-3 fatty acids, vitamin K, dietary fiber, and vitamin C and a good source of calcium and magnesium.

5. Fennel Seeds

In India Ayurvedic Physicians revered fennel seeds as digestive aid. It is still commonly being used there. Folk herbalists often mixed fennel with strong laxative herbs like senna and aloe to relieve the intestinal cramps that laxatives often cause. Fennel Seeds are included in the FDA's list of safe herbs. They are easily available in supermarkets.

In other countries fennel seeds are also used for indigestion, gas pain, irritable bowel syndrome and infant colic. Contemporary herbalists recommend fennel as a digestive aid, milk promoter, expectorant, eyewash and buffer in herbal laxative blends.

European research shows that fennel kills some bacteria, supporting the traditional role of fennel in treating diarrhea.

In many Indian restaurants you will find a bowl of plain or candied fennel seeds by the door as a digestive aid for departing diners. You can buy candied fennel seeds. Even children like them.

For women's health concerns fennel seeds were traditionally used as anti-spasmodic, to stimulate menstruation, and to relax the uterus. One study suggests that this herb also has a mild estrogenic effect. It means that fennel acts like the female sex hormone estrogen. Fennel seeds are still used in some cultures as milk producers and menstruation promoters. These seeds may help older women to relieve the discomforts of menopause.

Boil a spoonful of fennel seeds in 2 cups of water for 10 minutes, let it cool, strain and keep it in a clean bottle. Give ¼ to ½ spoon to babies and infants for digestion, gas and for diarrhea. It is commercially available in Indian subcontinent and in many European countries by the name of Gripe Water. Gripe water is an age-old remedy for colic that was traditionally made at home using dill, bicarbonate, and alcohol. Now, most drug stores carry commercially available gripe water but it does not contain alcohol.

These fennel seed based formulas may also include herbs that settle the stomach or help relax cramping muscles, such as ginger and dill. But it's important to recognize that gripe waters are not regulated by the Food and Drug Administration. Additionally, there is a small chance that your infant could be allergic to one or more of the ingredients. When first time administering it watch for any signs of allergic reactions.

For adults it is good for digestion, either chew a spoonful of fennel seeds or try an infusion or tincture. These infusions and tinctures are commercially available.

6.   Fenugreek Leaves and Seeds

Fenugreek is a small plant. Both the leaves and seeds are used in the kitchen of Indian sub-continent households. It is called "Methi". The seeds have a strong aroma and a bitter taste. But when used in small quantity they impart strong flavor to your food. It is commonly used in curries, vegetable dishes and lentils. Leaves are cooked as vegetables, alone or with potatoes. They are added to other vegetables for their aroma. They are also used in making a kind of flat bread called *methi paratha*.

Besides the use in kitchen *methi* is a rich reservoir of medicinal properties. *Methi* contains protein, fiber, vitamin C, niacin, potassium, iron and alkaloids. It also contains a compound that has diosgenin an oestrogen-like property, as well as steroidal saponins. Because of these compounds fenugreek or methi seeds are used in many beauty products and are the answer to many health problems! They are especially beneficial for women.

Fenugreek seeds are very beneficial for nursing mothers. This is due to the presence of diosgenin in the seeds that increases milk production in lactating mothers. Indian nursing women ate fenugreek seeds to increase their milk production. Arab women ate roasted seeds to help them gain weight, enlarge their breasts, and to attain plump and rounded figure.

Fenugreek seeds have been helpful in inducing childbirth by stimulating uterine contractions. It is also known to reduce labor pain. Fenugreek seeds are to be used in moderation. Excessive use during pregnancy could put you in risk of miscarriage or premature childbirth.

Though the leaves of fenugreek plant have medicinal value, the seeds have more potential in the treatment of certain conditions and diseases. Fenugreek is used for digestive problems such as loss of appetite, upset stomach, constipation, and inflammation of the stomach (gastritis). It is also used for conditions that affect heart health such as "hardening of the arteries" (atherosclerosis) and for high blood levels of certain fats including cholesterol and triglycerides.

Ancient physicians learned that fenugreek seeds contain a great deal of a special type of fiber called mucilage. When mixed with water mucilage becomes gelatinous and soothes inflamed or irritated tissue. In Ayurvedic medicine, these seeds are used as an herbal alternative to improve testosterone levels in men.

Egyptian physicians put fenugreek into ointments to treat wounds and abscesses. They also recommended using the herb internally to treat fevers and respiratory and intestinal complaints. Fenugreek is sometimes used as a poultice. That means it is wrapped in cloth, grinded warmed and applied directly to the skin to treat local pain and swelling muscle pain, pain and swelling of lymph nodes, pain in the toes (gout), wounds, leg ulcers, and eczema.

Modern herbalists recommend fenugreek poultices and plasters to treat wounds, boils and rashes.

Gargle with fenugreek seeds boiled in water, let it cool a little. It will soothe the sore throat. It has anti-inflammatory properties that may help in arthritis pain. Fenugreek seeds contain amino acids. The amino acid is useful in speeding up glycogen synthesis. Some bodybuilding products include this spice in their diet to help their body restores glycogen fast.

The seeds are also used in some cultures as a skin conditioner. The seeds are soaked in water and then applied on the skin. These seeds are also being used as a home remedy to prevent hair from falling out and thinning and may promote hair growth.

Fenugreek is available as whole dried seeds, fenugreek tea, tablets, capsules, fenugreek powder and liquid extract. You can make fenugreek tea by adding the seeds to hot water, sieve the seeds when it's cooled and drink it without adding any sweetener. You can add it to tea if you prefer. But as it is uterine stimulant pregnant women should not take it.

7. Garlic

Garlic is an herb. It is widely used around the world. It is best known for its pungent flavor as a seasoning or condiment. Its close relatives include the onion, shallot, leek and chive. Garlic is native to central Asia, and has been used for both culinary and medicinal purposes for years. But these days garlic is being used to treat a wide variety of diseases and conditions.

Garlic cloves have a characteristic pungent, spicy flavor that mellows and sweetens considerably with cooking. It is commonly used with onion, tomato and ginger, especially in meat dishes and sometimes in vegetarian dishes as well. Garlic leaves are a popular vegetable in many parts of Asia. The leaves are cut, cleaned, and then stir-fried with eggs, meat, or vegetables. Garlic powder is applied to different kinds of bread to create a variety of classic dishes, such as garlic bread, garlic toast. Some love to sprinkle garlic powder on pizza slices. Garlic powder has a different taste from fresh garlic. If used as a substitute for fresh garlic, 1/8 teaspoon of garlic powder is equivalent to one clove of garlic.

Oils can be flavored with garlic cloves. These infused oils are used to season all categories of vegetables, meats, breads and pasta.

Mixing garlic with egg yolks and olive oil produces *aioli*, a traditional sauce made of garlic, olive oil, lemon juice, and egg yolks.

Garlic, oil, and a chunky base produce a thick puree or sauce, dip, spread.

Blend garlic, almond, oil, and soaked bread. It produces *ajoblanco* a popular Spanish cold soup typical from Granada and Andalusia. This dish is made of bread, crushed almonds, garlic, water, olive oil, salt and sometimes vinegar. It is usually served with grapes or slices of melon.

Garlic is said to help regulate blood sugar levels. Regular and prolonged use of therapeutic amounts of aged garlic extracts lower blood homocysteine levels. Homocysteine is a naturally occurring amino acid found in blood plasma. High levels of homocysteine in the blood are believed to increase the chance of heart disease, stroke,

Aged garlic extracts help lower blood homocysteine levels, and has helped prevent diabetes mellitus. People taking insulin should not consume medicinal amounts of garlic without consulting a physician.

Garlic cloves are used as a remedy for infections (especially chest problems), digestive disorders, and fungal infections such as thrush. Garlic can be used as a disinfectant because of its bacteriostatic and bactericidal properties.

Garlic has been used reasonably successfully in AIDS patients to treat *Cryptosporidium* in an uncontrolled study in China. Some studies suggest that aged garlic extract can help in lowering systolic blood pressure similarly to current first line medications in patients with uncontrolled hypertension."

Research suggests that people who take a garlic supplement each day are more likely not to get cold. Although garlic has been traditionally used to fight off and treat the symptoms of the common cold, this is the first hard evidence of its medicinal properties. Garlic capsules are available that do not give the garlicky smell. These capsules are also being used for conditions like high blood pressure, high cholesterol, coronary heart disease, heart attack, and "hardening of the arteries". Garlic actually may be effective in slowing the development of atherosclerosis and seems to be able to modestly reduce blood pressure.

A large number of sulfur compounds contribute to the smell and taste of garlic. Abundant sulfur compounds in garlic are also responsible for turning garlic green or blue during pickling and cooking. Garlic is known for causing bad breath (halitosis), as well as causing sweat to have a pungent "garlicky" smell. Wash the skin with soap. Gargle with hydrogen peroxide to get rid of garlicky smell.

8. Ginger

Ginger is a plant that comes from Southeast Asia, and is now also cultivated in Jamaica and other tropical areas. Ginger is a natural spice and is known worldwide for its smell and pungent taste. Ginger has been used by Chinese herbalists for more than 2,500 years.

Ginger truly does top the list of effective natural home remedies. Being used throughout history by different cultures around the world, ginger has an incredible healing power proven for many ailments. It is packed with essential nutrients and rejuvenating compounds. Ginger is used in countless 'minor' problems such as an upset stomach. It's good to use ginger for nausea caused during pregnancy or by travelling.

Ginger calms an upset stomach and promotes the flow of bile.

Stomach cramps can be eased and circulation can also be improved with the use of ginger.

Ginger supports a healthy cardiovascular system by making platelets less sticky which in turn reduces circulatory problems.

In many herbal decongestants ginger is used to help minimize the symptoms of respiratory conditions, colds and allergies.

Ginger root is fast becoming a very popular medicinal herb.

Ginger root mixed with diluted lime juice can help to soothe the digestive tract and reduce flatulence.

Oil can be extracted from ginger which can be used to massage areas of localized chronic pain.

It can also be used to reduce inflammation as well.

Ginger tea can be taken several times a day. Crystallized ginger can be taken twice a day. It's like candy. A variety of ginger tea bags is available in the market.

With such a wide range ginger products available and with the ever increasing benefits of ginger being discovered ginger or a product of ginger is something that everyone should have in their homes.

There are no known drug side effects. Ginger does not interact with any other nutrients or drugs in the body and ginger in all forms is very safe to take.

Ginger capsules should be taken with a full glass of water or fluid. Ginger can be taken the day after surgery to prevent post surgery nausea but should be stopped at least three to four days prior to surgery, due to the fact that it can make blood platelets less sticky and therefore increases the risk of bleeding. For people undergoing radiotherapy or chemotherapy, ginger taken with food can help reduce stomach irritation.

People with gallstones should consult their doctors prior to taking ginger as it is known to increase bile flow.

Ginger is also one of the most famous natural cures for cough. Peel ginger, slice it or cut it into 1 inch pieces and boil it to ensure potency.

Drinking ginger as a tea will ease sore throat, non-stop coughing and even congestion. You may add honey or lemon to taste

Tea made with ginger is also great for cough, upset stomach, and headaches.

Try having some ginger tea with coconut milk and honey, it breaks up phlegm and gives a boost to the immune system.

Grate some ginger and pluck a few sprigs of mint leaves and steep in boiling water for a few minutes and enjoy with a spoonful of honey to subdue a bellyache. It's great for calming upset stomachs.

Herbs like peppermint, cayenne pepper and ginger can be beneficial in the treatment of headaches and migraines. To use the 3 herbs together in tea as a natural pain reliever, mix a one inch piece of ginger with a teaspoon of dried peppermint and a pinch of cayenne in boiling water. Sweeten only with honey and drink it.

People have been using ginger as a home remedy for toothaches from generations. Many people even experience immediate relief from the tooth pain. Rub raw ginger into the gums, or boil the ginger root, letting it cool and use it as a mouth rinse.

Ginger can also help with muscle soreness. Try some ginger tea after a workout.

Many branches of natural health care like herbal therapy, aroma therapy, ayurveda and naturopathy depend on the multiple ginger benefits.

People have been experiencing many health benefits of ginger for ages; it is time that you see it as more than just an ingredient for your dishes. Take it as a powerful natural remedy. Still do not depend on ginger for treatment of any serious diseases or conditions. See your doctor. Use ginger remedies only as supplements.

9. Green Tea

Tea has been cultivated for centuries, beginning in India and China. Today, tea is the most widely consumed beverage in the world, second only to water. Hundreds of millions of people drink tea.

In Far Eastern countries it's a practice to drink green tea after meals instead of juices and sodas as we do in the West. Especially when we are eating oily and fried meals cold sodas are not helping the stomach to function properly. Green tea or any other regular tea helps liquefying and digesting the food. It has its many more health benefits.

Green, black, and oolong tea are all derived from the leaves of the *Camellia sinensis* plant. Originally cultivated in East Asia, this plant grows as large as a shrub or tree. Today, *Camellia sinensis* grows throughout Asia and parts of the Middle East and Africa.

People in Asian countries more commonly consume green and oolong tea while black tea is most popular in the United States. Green tea is prepared from unfermented leaves, the leaves of oolong tea are partially fermented, and black tea is fully fermented. The more the leaves are fermented, the lower the polyphenol content (See: "What's It Made Of?") and the higher the caffeine content. Green tea has the highest polyphenol content while black tea has roughly 2-3 times the caffeine content of green tea.

The content of flavonoids in a cup of green tea is higher than that in the same volume of other food and drink items that are traditionally considered of health contributing nature, including fresh fruits, vegetable juices or wine. Among the young soda is the most popular beverage which is the most injurious drink for health. We constantly read the harms of drinking coco cola, pepsi etc.

Green tea has recently become more widespread in the West, where black tea has been the traditionally consumed tea.

Green tea has become the raw material for extracts which are used in various beverages, health foods, dietary supplements, and cosmetic items. Many varieties of green tea have been created in the countries where it is grown.

Green tea contains a variety of enzymes, amino acids, carbohydrates, lipids, sterols, polyphenols, carotenoids, tocopherols, vitamins, caffeine and related compounds, phytochemicals and dietary minerals. In traditional Chinese and Indian medicine, practitioners used green tea as a stimulant, a diuretic (to help rid the body of excess fluid), an astringent (to control bleeding and help heal wounds), and to improve heart health. Other traditional uses of green tea include treating gas, regulating body temperature and blood sugar, promoting digestion, and improving mental processes.

The Far East has been aware for centuries of the many health benefits associated with green tea extract. These benefits have now been backed by research, as it has been found that green tea extract is rich in polyphenols such as bioflavonoid and antioxidants. These fight free radicals present in the body. The antioxidant found in green tea is more effective in fighting free radicals than vitamins C and E.

White tea has anti-bacterial and anti-viral properties. Black tea can help lower blood pressure and prevent heart disease. Mint tea can also help treating bloating and aid digestion.

In traditional Chinese and Indian medicine, practitioners used green tea as a stimulant, a diuretic (to help rid the body of excess fluid), an astringent (to control bleeding and help heal wounds), and to improve heart health. Other traditional uses of green tea include treating gas, regulating body temperature and blood sugar, promoting digestion, and improving mental processes.

There are three main varieties of tea—green, black, and oolong. The difference is in how the teas are processed. Green tea is made from unfermented leaves and reportedly contains the highest concentration of powerful antioxidants called polyphenols.

Source: Green tea | University of Maryland Medical Center http://umm.edu/health/medical/altmed/herb/green-tea#ixzz2jV9sK4gA

10. Mint

Plants in the mint family are very hardy perennials with vigorous growth habits. Mint grows and spreads quickly. You only have to put a stem with roots in the soil and it will grow and spread quickly. It is easy to grow in a pot even indoors.

There are many varieties of mint, such as peppermint, apple mint, orange mint and curly mint. Each variety of mint has been used for culinary purposes and to cure numerous ailments, ranging from an upset stomach to nervousness.

In the home, mint has long been used as an aromatic herb. Today it is also commonly used in sachets and potpourris. Some soap makers add small amounts of dried mint to their soaps to make a cleansing soap for oily skin.

Many delicious meals are also flavored with mint. Favorite mint items include mint tea, mint sauce, and mint jelly. Mint leaves are also used to flavor cheeses, breads, and salads. Many Asian dishes, cool drinks and desserts are garnished with mint leaves. We can buy many things that are mint-flavored; cakes, meringues candies and cookies.

We can add it fresh to salads, soups, curry dishes and can make a marinade for lamb and other meats.

In Middle Eastern counties mint tea after meal is a popular drink. Add chopped mint to sauces for red meat particularly lamb.

Another Middle Eastern salad dish called Tabbouleh contains mint, bulgar, parsley, red onions, tomato and lemon juice and it is delicious.

Several sprigs of mint can be added to peas, green beans or new potatoes whilst boiling.

Mint is also added to a homemade or pre-prepared chocolate sauce for a choc and mint sauce.

You may like to make a yoghurt dressing with chopped mint leaves, garlic and salt and pepper for salads especially cucumber salad.

Add chopped mint to rice, chickpea, couscous or bean dishes for its flavor and aroma.

You may make a Mint Chutney to flavor veggies, fish, chicken, or lamb. We can dry mint leaves and save them to use in winter time.

Mint chutney: A bunch of mint leaves, ½ green bell pepper, 1 spoon cumin powder, juice of ½ lemon, and ½ spoon salt. Slightly coarsely blend all ingredients. Your mint chutney is ready.

Mix a tablespoon of mint chutney in a cup of yogurt and you have yogurt sauce. You may use it as a dip as well.

Add chopped mint to your ground meat dish, meat loaf, lentils. Garnish fish, steak and other meat dishes according to your taste.

The medicinal use of mint has been popular for ages to aid digestion and to relieve indigestion and heart burn. If you suffer from frequent indigestion, drinking a cup of peppermint tea after your meal may help.

Menthol is obtained from peppermint oil. It has healing properties and helps when rubbed on the chest to relieve the respiratory problems by opening the airways and respiratory passages.

Blend peppermint and tea tree oils, add Epsom salt and sea salts. Pour all ingredients in a bowl and add one liter of water. Mix well. Soak your feet. It will help eliminate fungus and bacteria from your feet and especially from your toe nails. It will leave your feet feeling soft, refreshed and odor free.

Mint's powerful antioxidants protect the body against the formation of cancerous cells. It also inhibits the growth of many different types of bacteria and fungus.

It helps to drink mint tea relieving the symptoms of colds and flu, nasal allergies congestion, headaches and head colds.

When you have minor aches and pains such as muscle cramps and sprains drinking mint tea will help relieve the pain.

Mint leaves provide a cooling sensation to the skin and can help to treat minor burns.

Mint tea can help clear up skin disorders such as acne.

11. Turmeric

Turmeric is a widely used tropical herb in the ginger cardamom and zedoary family. It's also known as Curcuma and Indian saffron. Its stalk is used both in food and medicine, yielding the familiar yellow ingredient that colors and adds flavor to. Turmeric is believed to strengthen the overall energy of the body, relieve gas, dispel worms, improve digestion, regulate menstruation, dissolve gallstones, and relieve arthritis, among other uses.

Indian researchers in 1971 found evidence suggesting that turmeric may possess anti-inflammatory properties. Curcumin is an antioxidant.

Turmeric's antioxidant abilities make it a good food preservative, provided that the food is already yellow in color, and it is widely used for this purpose.

Turmeric has been proposed as a treatment for dyspepsia. Dyspepsia includes a variety of digestive problems, such as stomach discomfort, gas, bloating, belching, appetite loss, and nausea. Although many serious medical conditions can cause digestive distress, the term dyspepsia is most often used when no identifiable medical cause can be detected.

Western science confirms that turmeric is a first rate anti-inflammatory herb. It contains at least two chemicals, curcumin and curcuminoids, that act to decrease inflammation linked to arthritic inflammation. This anti-inflammatory effect may be why consumption of turmeric is also connected to a reduced occurrence of cancers, cataracts and has been shown to be an effective pain reliever in cases of rheumatoid arthritis.

Modern studies confirm ancient wisdom that those with psoriasis can especially benefit from daily turmeric. Studies show that the curcumin in turmeric acts to disrupt the cycle of skin plaque formation.

It is a useful in dental and oral care treatment because of its medicinal properties such as anti-inflammatory, antioxidant, and antimicrobial activity. In a recent study turmeric mouthwash (10 mg curcumin extract dissolved in 100 ml of water with a peppermint flavoring agent added) was found to be as effective as a solution made from chlorhexidine gluconate (CHX), the gold standard compound for plaque buildup in dentistry.

This is a healthy and inexpensive spice and is great for cooking, and it may help to limit weight gain from a high fat diet. It has almost no side effects except for the people with hypoglycemia. Small amount of turmeric in cooking is fine but should not take large amounts.

Turmeric is a mild aromatic stimulant used in manufacturing of curry powders and mustards. Used as a "poor persons" saffron to color rice. It should be taken as daily supplement and used as healthy culinary spice. Turmeric is the best medicine in Ayurveda. It cures the whole person. Turmeric is pungent and bitter. The yellow color of turmeric can stain clothes and skin.

Turmeric can be applied topically to a painful joint or swelling as a poultice to relieve pain.

You may add half tea spoon of turmeric powder to milk and take it in the night at bed time, especially women after child birth.

Turmeric roots look like ginger roots but a little smaller. Peel and slice them and add in salads, soups (will color it yellow) and to certain meat dishes.

You may take turmeric in supplement form in order to reap the medicinal benefits.

Chapter 6

OILS AND OTHER PRODUCTS

1. Castor Oil

Plant-based castor oil has gained popularity for its various applications. The oil is found in the soaps you lather on your skin, the inks you use for printing and the plastic goods you use every day. Unlike other vegetable oils with limited applications, it plays a notable role in conventional medicine and in the industrial world, among many other areas.

Castor oil has been ignored by modern medicine despite a centuries old history of medicinal uses. It has been used as a laxative or purging cleanse and parasite remover for years. Castor oil packs applied externally can go beyond skin care to affect internal organs beneath epidermal application as well.

Castor oil is one of the oldest treatments for aging skin. In Egypt the ancient Pharaohs used castor oil on their skin. In modern times it is a popular ingredient in commercial skin moisturizers and other products. These products are effective for anti-aging treatment and for wrinkles and are also affordable options available.

Castor oil moisturizes skin, prevents dryness and makes it look younger and fresh. Dryness causes skin to look aged and wrinkled after certain age. Castor oil improves the circulation of the skin. Improved blood flow allows the skin to get more oxygen and nutrients which help to prevent the signs of aging.

When you are using cold pressed castor oil, there are antioxidants available to fight free radicals in the skin cells, thus castor oil is a great way to reduce and prevent wrinkles.

Edgar Cayce, who authored the Encyclopedia of Healing, said that castor oil supported the healing of the small intestines, particularly the lymphatic tissue—this allowed for tissue growth and repair.

Naturopathic practitioners claim that castor oil helps strengthen the immune system.

As a laxative, a teaspoon or so works well taken before bed for morning constipation relief. Castor oil can be used topically for skin problems ranging from fungal toenails to acne. Castor oil is anti-fungal and anti-viral. Castor oil is also considered to be good for your hair.

Medicinal castor oil should never be used by pregnant women. There is a risk of induced abortion.

2.   Coconut Oil

Coconut oil is best for hair care. Massage with it and leave it for at least one hour then wash your hair. Coconut oil will leave your hair silky, sleek and smooth.

It is good for skin care. Massage your face, arms and whole body with it. It will take care of your skin, will have no blemishes. Skin will be soft and sooth.

It will also give relief from stress.

Cooking with coconut oil will maintain your cholesterol levels. As a matter of fact it will help you lose weight. It will increase immunity, help in proper digestion and metabolism. It is also good for kidney problems and heart diseases, high blood pressure and diabetes. Take a piece of fresh coconut and eat it after every meal. It is good for dental care and also for bone strengthening.

Cook your meals in coconut oil. Use it for hair and skin care. Use it to maintain cholesterol, kidneys, high blood pressure and diabetes.

Use a teaspoon after every meal to increase immunity, metabolism and digestion.

Eat raw coconut for dental care.

For detailed information on coconut please read Chapter 2.

3.   Olive Oil

Olive oil is a fat obtained from the fruit of the olive tree, a traditional tree crop of the Mediterranean region, where whole olives are pressed to produce olive oil. The health benefits, as well as the wonderful flavor and taste of olive oil on salads, pasta, fish and almost in anything has known to Mediterranean people. Fortunately it is available all over the world throughout the year for everyone to satisfy taste buds and promote good health.

Homer referred to olive oil as liquid gold, and Thomas Jefferson proclaimed it the richest gift of heaven. For centuries, this gift of olive oil was always a welcome treasure. But in recent years there is a new awareness of the benefits of olive oil and it has become part of many more households. Besides cooking it is being used for healing and curing purposes. It is also being used in many beauty products, like soaps, moisturizers etc. Nature has provided dietary fats in the olive oil exactly as much as needed in the human body to maintain good health. Some cardiologists recommend at least two tablespoons of extra virgin olive oil each day to enjoy the full benefits of olive oil to your heart health and well being. Virgin means made with physical processes, not using any chemical processes. Extra virgin is the highest quality and most expensive olive oil. It should have no defects and should have a flavor of fresh olives. Essentially crush an olive and out drop the oil in extreme synthesis.

Olive oil helps lower levels of blood cholesterol which is a leading cause of heart disease. Olive oil intake (about 4 spoons a day) is associated with decreased risk of heart disease, stroke or dying of heart disease, according to the recent study published in the New England Journal of Medicine.

Did you know something? About Olive it's mentioned in couple of the verses in the Holy Book Al-Qur'an.

". . . it from a blessed tree, an olive, neither of the east nor of the west, its oil all but giving off light even if no fire touches it. Light upon Light. Allah guides to His Light whoever He wills and Allah makes metaphors for mankind and Allah has knowledge of all things." (Qur'an, 24:35)

"And by it He makes crops grow for you and olives and dates and grapes and fruit of every kind. There is certainly a Sign in that for people who reflect." (Qur'an, 16:11)

Numerous studies have only reinforced the notion that olive oil is an amazing substance with numerous benefits. Here are 101 of them.

Olive oil can:

1. Make your arteries more elastic—Two tablespoons daily makes you more resistant to strokes and heart attack.
2. Reduce bad cholesterol levels—Olive oil contains polyphenols, which help to keep your levels of LDL cholesterol within healthy ranges.
3. Make you less hungry—Olive oil makes you feel sated and tends to make you eat less and have fewer sugar cravings.
4. Reduce the risk of stroke in the elderly through yet another mechanism—Older people who ate diets rich in olive oil

consumption, which contains plasma oleic acid, had fewer strokes in a 2011 study.

5. Lower the risk of coronary heart disease in women—Mediterranean cultures have long revered the olive and its oil, with good reason. An Italian study found that a diet that included olive oil along with plenty of leafy vegetables and fruit resulted in reduced rates of coronary heart disease in women enrolled in the study.

6. Cure or reduce acne—Although it sounds counterintuitive to use oil to fight pimples and blackheads, using an olive oil and salt scrub helps some types of acne.

7. Protect your red blood cells and therefore your heart—Over time, cells oxidize, leading to the common effects of aging. A specific polyphenol in olive oil is especially effective at protecting your red blood cells from oxidation. A 2009 study identified this component as DHPEA-EDA.

8. Treat sunburn—Olive oil soothes the pain of mild sunburn by helping skin retain its moisture. Use equal parts olive oil and water in a tight-lidded container. Shake well, then apply to mild sunburn. Shake the mixture often during application to keep it from separating.

9. Help fight breast cancer—Olive oil contains phytochemicals, and a 2008 study found that they are effecting at killing cancer cells and suppressing cancer genes.

10. Improve your memory—Some research has shown that olive oil can prevent and possibly even reverse the memory loss that accompanies Alzheimer's disease.

11. Prevent heart attacks in men—A 2008 study showed that men who ate at least two ounces of olive oil reduced their chances of having a heart attack by 82 percent as compared to men who ate no olive oil.

12. Keep your lips soft and supple—Make your own lip balm by combining olive oil with equal parts beeswax. Put it into a small glass jar and apply it with your fingertip.

13. Condition your hair—Ancient beauties and warriors alike used olive oil to tame and beautify their locks. Olive oil strengthens hair and makes it more flexible.

14. Help you to stay healthier into old age—The Mediterranean Diet has been proven to be one of the healthiest in the world. Some consider it the healthiest. Olive oil has always been an integral part of the Mediterranean Diet. Although red wine and lots of fish, whole grains, fruits and vegetables also play a

huge part in the diet's success, scientists agree that it wouldn't be nearly as beneficial without olive oil.

15. Prevent dry scalps—Using olive oil as a scalp conditioner moisturizes your dry scalp.

16. Prevent middle-age spread—Because olive oil is a calorie-dense food, it is often avoided out of fear that it will cause weight gain. However, a 2008 study showed that olive oil, along with nut oils, did not cause weight gain the way less healthy fats do.

17. Provide an easy way to add minimally processed food to your diet—Extra virgin olive oil (EVOO) is unrefined. It is obtained by pressing cold olives. All other oils that are readily available to consumers must be refined using heat and other harsh processes.

18. Clean sensitive skin—The Ancient Egyptians, Greeks and Romans had no soap and didn't miss it thanks to olive oil. They massaged olive oil into their skin, then scraped it back off, along with dirt and dead skin. Today, a wide variety of soaps, including some made from olive oil, are available. Yet many people still prefer to clean their skin with pure olive oil.

19. Remove paint from your skin—Olive oil gently loosens paint on your skin. When you wipe away the oil, the paint goes with it. Your skin will be left soft, firm and smooth.

20. Make an inexpensive exfoliant that works like the most expensive spa products available—Exfoliating removes dead skin and prevents your skin from becoming dull. Mix a palmful of olive oil with a teaspoon of sugar or salt. Apply the mixture to your skin, then massage gently.

21. Moisturize your skin—Olive oil is closer in chemical structure to your skin's natural oil than any other naturally occurring oil. Use it as you would a body, face and hand lotion.

22. Prevent your skin from aging prematurely—The same antioxidant properties that keep your red blood cells from oxidizing when you eat olive oil keep your skin cells from oxidizing when you apply it topically. The antioxidant hydroxytyrosol and vitamin E help to prevent cell degeneration in your skin.

23. Never clog your pores or cause pimples—Olive oil penetrates the skin, leaving your skin silky smooth with no greasy feeling. Cleopatra undoubtedly had many costly beauty secrets up her sleeve, but the most important of them can be yours for the price of a small bottle of EVOO.

24. Prevent sagging skin—The squalene in olive oil increases your skin's elasticity, leaving it firmly toned with a bright, youthful glow.

25. Smooth and moisturize rough, dry feet—Make a foot scrub of equal parts olive oil and honey, a third part sugar and a dash of lemon juice. Soak your feet in warm water, then massage the moisture into them. Follow up by moisturizing your feet and hands with a well-shaken water and olive oil emulsion.

26. Give you a safe sunless tan—Use olive oil as a medium to make self-tanners go on more smoothly and evenly. Mix equal parts of a commercial self-tanning product and olive oil. Apply the mixture to your skin and enjoy your streak-free sunless tan.

27. Act as a perfect medium for cosmetics—Combined with natural pigments and beeswax, olive oil makes inexpensive, natural lip-gloss, blush and even eye shadow.

28. Make a perfect addition to homemade skin-care products—Nearly all your skin-care recipes, from masks to exfoliants, can be improved by substituting olive oil for the oil called for in the original recipe. You can also often improve and extend expensive commercial skin care products by mixing a small amount with a palmful of olive oil just before you use them.

29. Act as a perfect carrier for oil-based medicines—Essential oils usually cannot be used full-strength on the skin. They typically require the use of a carrier oil. Olive oil is excellent carrier oil for most essential oils.

30. Team up with mashed avocado for a homemade facial mask—Mix olive oil with a mashed ripe avocado into a paste. Smooth onto your face or another area that needs moisturizing and rejuvenating. Allow to sit for 15 minutes, then rinse.

31. Combine with honey and egg for a beauty mask right from the pages of Venus' beauty guide—An ancient beauty mask recipe is made from an egg yolk, a spoonful of honey and a spoonful of olive oil. Rub it on and wait for 15 minutes, then rinse it all off with warm water.

32. Make a natural vitamin supplement—Two tablespoons can replace your daily vitamin E supplement while providing all the other benefits of olive oil.

33. Possibly protect and lubricate your voice—There is no scientific evidence yet to back them up, but singers have been using olive oil as a gargle before performing for centuries.

34. Make a natural massage oil—Olive oil may very well be the world's oldest massage oil. It can be used alone or as a carrier

oil for essential oils. Learn about why olive oil is great for massage.

35. Enhance spirituality—Homer makes reference to the use of olive oil as an anointing oil. In ancient times, anointing was very important. Olive oil was often combined with myrrh or cinnamon oil before it was used for this sacred purpose.

36. Improve your skin's appearance from the inside out—Including olive oil in your daily diet helps your skin stay healthy and beautiful.

37. Act as an all-natural personal lubricant—Olive oil is almost certainly the world's oldest personal lubricant. It should not be used in combination with latex condoms or diaphragms, however.

38. Help fight off degenerative diseases—The antioxidants in olive oil give it the power to help lessen the impact of degenerative diseases on your body.

39. Improve the health of the entire population of the world—The World Health Organization officially recommends that people across the world adopt the Mediterranean diet for better health and specifically suggests olive oil as the healthiest source of fat on the planet.

40. Hold its own next to fruits and vegetables as a source of antioxidants and vitamins—EVOO is a natural, minimally processed food that contains as many antioxidants and nutrients as many foods that are touted as health foods.

41. Lower your blood pressure—Although researchers have some theories as to why it works, no one is sure why olive oil helps to lower blood pressure. They just know that it does.

42. Reduce nitric acid to normal levels—Nitric acid has been proven to increase blood pressure. Olive oil reduces nitric acid levels. This may be one of the ways it lowers your blood pressure.

43. Take the credit for making women beautiful—The Bible mentions that the Persian king Xerxes' wives used olive oil to make themselves beautiful. More recently, Sophia Loren, who is still being named to "most beautiful" lists in her 70s, credits her beauty to olive oil baths. She also claims to consume olive oil daily.

44. Make fine soap—The very first soap in the world was made of olive oil. Today, olive oil soap is still one of the smoothest, best-smelling soaps on the market.

45. Combine with butter for a healthier bread spread—In a mixing bowl, combine one part softened butter and one part olive oil. Mix on low until the oil is whipped into the butter. Refrigerate and use it as you would butter.

46. Make you live longer—There is no doubt that eating a healthy diet can make you live longer. Olive oil is part of the healthiest diet on earth, the Mediterranean Diet. Jeanne Calment, who currently has the distinction of being the longest-living person whose age could be confirmed in the world, needed no convincing. She lived to be a very youthful 122 and gave the credit to her daily consumption of olive oil. She also used it topically.

47. Minimize cellulite—Mix used coffee grounds with olive oil for a topical cellulite treatment. Apply it directly to the skin.

48. Help you get a sunless tan without using commercial products—If you don't like the thought of mixing olive oil with a commercial self-tanning lotion, mix it with used coffee grounds instead. Apply it liberally but evenly in the tub before your shower and allow it to work its magic.

49. Condition your hair—Used coffee grounds and olive oil make a good hair conditioner, as well. Rub it in well before you shampoo your hair.

50. Deep condition damaged hair—Warm a quarter cup of olive oil to a comfortable temperature, then work it through your hair to the roots. Wrap your hair in plastic wrap or a shower cap, then heat your hair with a hair dryer. Allow the oil to sit on your hair for up to a half hour, then shampoo as usual. If you do this in the shower, your whole body will emerge soft and silky.

51. Remove makeup—Apply olive oil to a cotton ball and gently wipe your makeup off your face. You can safely use olive oil near your eyes.

52. Firm and tone skin—Combine equal parts water and olive oil in a jar or other container with a tight-fitting lid. Shake well. Apply to your skin.

53. Add a new dimension to ordinary wrestling matches—In Turkey, a 600-year-old tradition involves grown men wrestling while covered in olive oil.

54. Act as a sensual massage oil—Olive oil has been used as a sensual massage oil since ancient times.

55. Help you create delicious, healthy baked goods—Olive oil is commonly used in baking in the Mediterranean. Use a

lighter-colored, lighter tasting end-of-season version for desserts.

56. Ensure your baked goods come out of the pan in one piece—Olive oil can be rubbed or misted on baking pans instead of baking sprays or shortening.

57. Turn fast food into health food—Use olive oil to transform unhealthy American pizza into healthy Mediterranean pizza by substituting it for other oils and using it to oil the pan and shine up the finished crust.

58. Keep baked goods fresh longer—The vitamin E in olive oil helps to keep baked goods moist and fresh longer than solid shortenings or even other oils.

59. Replace butter in recipes—Olive oil is a good substitute for butter in recipes. It even works in baked goods. Use slightly less than the amount of butter called for in the recipe.

60. Return Italian dishes to their healthy roots—Use olive oil in sauces, to prevent pasta from sticking and to sauté ingredients. A little of the right oil can make the difference between a health dish and an unhealthy one.

61. Make heaven on a plate—Make heart-healthy pesto by grinding basil, walnuts or pine nuts, parmesan and garlic together, then incorporating EVOO until the texture is right. Serve over pasta or as a dipping sauce for bread.

62. Protect food from freezer burn—Use as a protective seal for homemade sauces or other Mediterranean dishes before you freeze them.

63. Prevent mosquitoes from breeding—Prevent mosquito larvae from contaminating rainwater by pouring a layer of olive oil on top of the water in your rain barrel.

64. Make a heart-healthy condiment—EVOO is delicious drizzled over bread and many other dishes.

65. Make a heart-healthy salad dressing—Combine equal parts EVOO and balsamic vinegar, raspberry vinegar or red wine vinegar and drizzle over your salad.

66. Make ordinary bread something special—Bread dipping oils can be flavored with a variety of herbs and spices. Start with EVOO and use your imagination.

67. Combine with herbs, spices, garlic or citrus juices to make your taste buds pop—Infuse EVOO with herbs for dipping sauces. Experiment with adding garlic alone or in combination with herbs, spices, vinegars or lemon or other citrus juices.

68. Compliment or contrast with your food—Different EVOOs pair beautifully with foods. Choose flavors of EVOO that either compliment or contrast with the food you are serving it with, then drizzle the cold oil over the food.
69. Reduce the appearance of stretch marks—Combine equal parts cocoa butter and olive oil for a stretch-mark minimizer.
70. Enhance the beauty of black hair—Combine olive oil with hair care products to make the product spread more evenly through your hair.
71. Detangle your hair—Work olive oil into your hair, then comb the tangles right out of it.
72. Shine and seal your hair—After moisturizing, apply olive oil to prevent the moisture from evaporating.
73. Boost a commercial conditioner—Add olive oil to conditioner to enhance and improve it.
74. Prevent hair loss and damage—By using olive oil to manage your hair instead of using harsh chemicals, you can minimize damage to your hair.
75. Kill lice—To kill lice, follow the directions for using olive oil as a deep conditioning treatment. Make sure to leave the oil on your child's hair for at least 30 minutes and repeat the treatment every ten days for at least a month.
76. Prevent prematurely gray hair—EVOO contains pigments. Using it in your hair will gradually darken it.
77. Aid digestion—People have taken olive oil as a digestive aid for generations.
78. Make a sweet-smelling, clean-burning lamp oil—Olive oil lamps have been prized for thousands of years for their good light and lack of sputter.
79. Act as a household lubricant—Use olive oil anywhere you would use a lubricant spray or 3in1 oil.
80. Shine household surfaces—Appliances, faucets, stainless steel and laminate surfaces all benefit from a light coating of olive oil and a gentle buffing.
81. Condition cutting boards—Rub olive oil lightly on cutting boards, wooden salad bowls and wooden utensils.
82. Sauté food—You can sauté most foods in olive oil. Avoid high heat and don't try to use it for deep-frying.
83. Darken and highlight eyelashes—Use olive oil instead of mascara to darken and shine your eyelashes and eyebrows.

84. Turn or bath into a spa—Add olive oil to your bath the way you would use any bath oil. Experiment with using different essential oils to scent it.

85. Soothe a baby's delicate skin—Use olive oil instead of baby oil for baby care, especially to treat and prevent diaper rash.

86. Waterproof your work boots—It also works on tool belts, baseball gloves and other utilitarian leather items.

87. Smooth out that rough shave—Use olive oil instead of soap or shaving cream for a close, comfortable shave.

88. Polish wood furniture—Apply olive oil to a soft cloth, then wipe it onto your furniture.

89. Condition cuticles—Apply olive oil on a cotton swab to moisturize your cuticles.

90. Keep measuring cups clean—Wipe measuring containers with olive oil to allow sticky ingredients to slide right out of the pan.

91. Tame frizzy hair—Lightly spray olive oil on frizzy hair before combing.

92. Unstick a zipper—Allow oil to penetrate the zipper, then unzip as usual.

93. Improve a cat's coat—Add a small amount of olive oil to cat food for a shinier coat and healthy skin.

94. Lend a shine to brass—Apply olive oil to a soft cloth, then rub it onto brass hardware.

95. Ease earache pain—A popular over-the-counter earache remedy has only one ingredient: olive oil.

96. Ease a scratchy throat tickle—A sip of EVOO may quiet that annoying tickle.

97. Make shoes shine—Lightly dampen a soft cloth with olive oil, then buff your shoes with it.

98. Protect hands from yard work—Put olive oil on your hands before gardening or other dirty work to prevent dirt buildup and make cleanup easier.

99. Remove sap or tar from your skin—Apply olive oil to the sticky spot, then rub gently until the residue is removed. Wipe the oil off your hands.

100. Remove stickers—Saturate the sticker with olive oil, then gently peel it off the surface.

101. Remove chewing gum from skin or non-porous surfaces— Rub the gum gently with olive oil. It might also help you pass chewing gum you have swallowed, but consult a doctor if you have swallowed more than a piece or two.

This information about the benefits of olive oil is included in my book with the permission of Dr. Robbins' response.

Hi Shamim

Thank you for your email. It would be our pleasure to have you include our information.

Best
Robbie Robbins M.D., D.D.S. FAAOHNS
Robbins Family Farm

4. Baking Soda

There are many uses of baking soda beside cleaning and deodorizing. It must be in every household.

- Soda absorbs radiation, absorbs heavy metals, and alkalizes the body.
- Baking soda may be used as tooth paste and mouth freshener.
- We can use it to wash dishes, clean floors, furniture and shower curtains.
- We can clean baby clothes and cloth diapers.
- Soda can be used as facial scrub and body exfoliant and as a non-toxic deodorant.
- You can treat itchy skin and insect bites with baking soda.
- Make a soak bath and soothe your feet; make a cleanser and softener, and deodorize stinky feet.
- You can also clean your bathroom tubs, tiles and sinks.
- Baking soda can be used for cleaning batteries and cars.
- Freshen up your linen with it.
- Use it to clean brushes and combs.
- Treat colds and flu.

In the kitchen use it to wash and clean dirt and residue off fresh fruits and vegetables.

5. Honey

Honey is one of nature's most versatile foods. It not only serves as a delicious, all-natural sweetener, but it's a helpful tool in supporting a healthy body and glowing appearance. No wonder it's been so popular for thousands of years and has been used all over the world by all cultures. Even in USA by American Indians honey was used as a fruit preservative and base for many herbal medicines. Adults and children love it alike. Make a peanut butter and honey (instead of jelly) sandwich for children and they will be delighted with it. Spread honey on flat bread, roll it and enjoy a delicious snack. Add honey to tea instead of sugar if you are diabetic. Add honey and ice to milk and you have an instant cold drink in summer.

Scientists of today also note honey as very effective medicine for all kinds of diseases. Honey can be used without side effects which is also a plus. Today's science says that even though honey is sweet, when it is taken in the right dosage as a medicine, it does not harm even diabetic patients.

Centuries ago in the Holy Book Quran it was declared that there is cure and healing in honey. "There comes forth from their bellies a drink of varying color wherein is healing for people. Verily, in this is indeed a sign for the people who think." Quran 16:69

Honey is antibacterial, antiseptic, antifungal, immune system booster, increases energy and stamina and is cough suppressant. Honey should be in every household.

Honey is considered the best remedy for diarrhea when mixed in hot water. It is the food of foods, drink of drinks and drug of drugs. It is used for creating appetite, strengthening the stomach, eliminating phlegm; as a meat preservative, hair conditioner, eye soother and mouthwash. It is extremely beneficial in the morning in warm water.

Honey can promote relaxation and help ease you to sleep at night.

Take half a lemon and put 3 or 4 drops of honey on it. Rub the lemon on all over your face. Leave it for five minutes and then wash it with cold water. It will leave your skin soft and moisturized. It will also fade other marks and spots from your face.

To make a wonderful remedial drink you need one beet root, one carrot and one apple and combine together. Peel the skin, cut into pieces and put them into the juicer. Add a spoon of honey and drink immediately.

You can add some lime or lemon for more refreshing taste. This wonderful drink will be an effective remedy for the eyesight. It will eliminate red and tired eyes or dry eyes. It will make skin healthy and look more radiant. This drink will detoxify your system, assist bowel movement and eliminate constipation. This drink will also help prevent liver, kidney, pancreas disease and it can cure ulcer as well. It will improve bad breath due to indigestion, as well as throat infection and pain. This drink will be a good remedy for Hay Fever.

A mixture of honey and Cinnamon cures many diseases. Make a paste of honey and cinnamon powder, put it on toast instead of jelly and jam and eat it regularly for breakfast. It reduces the cholesterol and could potentially save one from heart attack. Also, even if you have already had an attack studies show you could be kept miles away from the next attack. Regular use of cinnamon honey strengthens the heart beat.

In America and Canada, various nursing homes have treated patients successfully and have found that as one ages the arteries and veins lose their flexibility and get clogged; honey and cinnamon revitalize the arteries and the veins.

Arthritis patients can benefit by taking one cup of hot water with two tablespoons of honey and one small teaspoon of cinnamon powder. When taken daily even chronic arthritis can be cured. In a recent research conducted at the Copenhagen University, it was found that when the doctors treated their patients with a mixture of one tablespoon Honey and half teaspoon Cinnamon powder before breakfast, they found that within a week (out of the 200 people so treated) practically 73 patients were totally relieved of pain—and within a month, most all the patients who could not walk or move around because of arthritis started walking without pain.

Take two tablespoons of cinnamon powder and one teaspoon of honey in a glass of lukewarm water and drink it. It destroys the germs in the bladder. Constant use of Honey strengthens the white blood corpuscles (where DNA is contained) to fight bacterial and viral diseases.

One spoon of honey and one spoon of Cinnamon Powder added to a tall cup of tea drunk daily will reduce the level of cholesterol in the blood by 10 percent, and will also cure the arthritis pain.

In common or severe colds one should take one tablespoon lukewarm honey with 1/4 spoon cinnamon powder daily for three days. This will cure most chronic cough, cold, and, clear the sinuses, and it's delicious.

Honey taken with cinnamon powder cures stomach ache and also is said to clear stomach ulcers from its root.

According to the studies done in India and Japan, it is revealed that when Honey is taken with cinnamon powder the stomach is relieved of gas.

Apply honey and cinnamon powder in equal parts on the affected parts cures eczema, ringworm and all types of skin infections.

Daily in the morning one half hour before breakfast and on an empty stomach, and at night before sleeping, drink honey and cinnamon powder boiled in one cup of water. When taken regularly, it reduces the weight of even the most obese person.

Recent studies have shown that the sugar content of honey is more helpful rather than being detrimental to the strength of the body. Senior citizens who take honey and cinnamon powder in equal parts are more alert and flexible.

Dr. Milton, who has done research, says that a half tablespoon of honey taken in a glass of water and sprinkled with cinnamon powder, even when the vitality of the body starts to decrease, when taken daily after brushing and in the afternoon at about 3:00 P.M., the vitality of the body increases within a week.

So you see honey is a must in every household, as a food, as a drink, and as a medicine.

6. Hydrogen Peroxide

Hydrogen peroxide is the only germicidal agent composed only of water and oxygen. It kills disease organisms and microorganisms by oxidation. Hydrogen peroxide is considered the world's safest and natural effective sanitizer. When Hydrogen peroxide reacts with organic material it breaks down into oxygen and water.

An alternative to bleach hydrogen peroxide can be used to whiten the clothes. Add a cup of peroxide to white clothes in your laundry to whiten them. Peroxide is great to get rid of blood stains on clothes and carpets. If there is blood on clothing, just pour it directly on the spot, let it sit for about a minute, then rub and rinse with cold water. Repeat if blood I stain is old. Wash the clothing with cold water and soap after removing the peroxide treated blood.

It is also used to bleach human hair. The chemical's bleaching property lends its name to the phrase "peroxide blonde". When hydrogen peroxide is used to bleach the skin it is absorbed by skin upon contact and creates a local skin capillary embolism that appears as a temporary whitening of the skin. Hydrogen peroxide mixed with baking soda and salt is used as toothpaste.

Mixed with baking soda and a small amount of hand soap, hydrogen peroxide is effective at removing skunk odor. Hydrogen peroxide can be used to clean tile and grout on floors. It is sometimes recommended to clean with both hydrogen peroxide and baking soda together.

Hydrogen peroxide must be kept in every ones bathroom or medicine cabinet. It makes a very effective and inexpensive mouthwash.

To cure a foot fungus, simply spray a 50/50 mixture of Hydrogen peroxide and water on toes every night and let dry.

If your house is water damaged for any reason and becomes a biohazard if it's invaded by toxic mold then clean it with hydrogen peroxide.

As it is non-toxic, you can use it to disinfect fruits and vegetables, as well as pet toys, equipment and cages.

Hydrogen peroxide is generally recognized as safe as an antimicrobial agent, and an oxidizing agent. For example, 35% hydrogen peroxide is used to prevent infection transmission in the hospital environment, and hydrogen peroxide vapor is registered with the US EPA as a sporicidal sterilant.

Concentrated hydrogen peroxide (>50%) is corrosive, and even domestic-strength solutions can cause irritation to the eyes, mucous membranes and skin. Swallowing hydrogen peroxide solutions is particularly dangerous, as decomposition in the stomach releases large quantities of gas (10 times the volume of a 3% solution) leading to internal bleeding. Inhaling over 10% can cause severe pulmonary irritation.

Hydrogen peroxide should be stored in a cool, dry, well-ventilated area and away from any flammable or combustible substances.

7. Listerine

Listerine is a brand of antiseptic mouthwash product. It helps prevent cavities. It freshens the breath, kills the bad odor in the mouth. Listerine also strengthens teeth and restores minerals to enamel. It also cleans the whole mouth. It "kills germs that cause bad breath",

The ingredients found in Listerine, including eucalyptus, alcohol and thyme can kill bacteria that cause acne. Simply dab Listerine on the affected area using a clean cotton ball, and skip the pricey products. Just be sure not to use too much, and be cautious if you have sensitive skin.

Listerine is great for killing germs, which is why we use it. So you may clean your toothbrush with Listerine after each brushing.

Listerine is actually made with anti-fungal ingredients; it makes a great remedy for dandruff. For dandruff treatment use Listerine. Wet your hair thoroughly with the mouthwash and wrap your hair in a towel. After15 minutes shampoo as normal. You may need to do multiple treatments to get rid of the dandruff completely.

To eliminate sink odors, simply pour half a cup of mouthwash down the disposal.

You can also use Listerine as a deodorant. Simply dab a bit of the mouthwash on a cotton ball or towel, wipe it on your underarms.

Because Listerine kills odors and disinfects, it is a great for general cleaning. You can use it to clean toilets, sinks and floors.

To make a Vinegar and Listerine Foot Soak take 1 cup Listerine, 1 cup white vinegar, and 4 cups of warm water to be mixed together. Pour it in a big basin or in the tub. Soak your feet in this mixture for 20 to 30 minutes, the dead skin on your feet would just wipe right off. You may also use pumice stone to remove the calluses. The minty smell of the Listerine will leave feet smelling pretty good all day.

Listerine contains essential oils including thymol, eucalyptol, menthol and methyl salicylate. It also has 26.9 percent alcohol, which may kill lice.

8. Petroleum Jelly

Petroleum jelly jar is probably found in every household. You can do so many jobs with petroleum jelly instead of buying expensive products. It's cheap and easily available.

On your dry and chapped heels use a lot of jelly at night, cover your heel with a non-absorbing paper and put on your sock to keep the jelly and paper on your heel. Use a few times and your heels will be soft and smooth.

Highlight cheekbones. Fake a model's bone structure by patting and blending a tiny amount across cheekbones. The shine attracts light and creates a contoured effect.

Mix petroleum jelly and a little bit of coarse chick pea (beson) flour and buff away your dry skin. Wash it with warm water.

If you want to give shine and wet look to your lips use jelly instead of any lips gloss. You may add red or any food color of your choice.

Get an even tan. Dry skin tends to soak up excess tanning lotion, leaving skin splotchy. Smooth on petroleum jelly before using tanning products.

Preserve your fragrance. Dab on pulse points, like your wrists and the sides of your neck, before spraying on perfume. Your scent will last the entire day.

Use it as eye makeup remover. Take your finger tip take a little bit of jelly, apply it on your eye lid and then gently remove your make up with a tissue.

Smooth a layer at your hairline before using home color and you'll avoid hard-to-remove dark stains.

Coat ends to conceal dryness and frizz when you're between trims. You can also rub a little between your hands and use as hair wax for texture or to smooth flyaways. Wash it out.

Running low on your favorite moisturizer? Add petroleum jelly to prolong its life.

Dab a little petroleum jelly around your nails when you're having a manicure or pedicure done to keep polish from getting on your skin.

Before going to bed, rub petroleum jelly on places where skin is extra-dry, like on your elbows or the heels of your feet. Use a few days and the skin of your elbows and heel will be super-soft again. I have always used it on my heels especially in winter.

If your ring is stuck on your finger petroleum jelly can help it slide off easily.

Apply petroleum jelly to squeaky hinges on doors or cabinets to keep them quiet.

Petroleum jelly can make leather shoes shine like new again.

Chapter 7

LIVING HEALTHY

Eat Healthy Food and Stay in Good Health

In this chapter all the recipes of exotic healthy foods are given. Some recipes are my own age-old family recipes. Some I have created myself. In these recipes best quality of herbs and spices is used. Try to include some of them according to your taste and choices in your daily diet.

1. Recipes of Soups

Soups are so hearty, filling and delicious and at the same time so nutritious that they are full meals in themselves. You may drink your soup or make it thick enough to eat. Serve them with different kinds of breads with butter or cheese, with rice, pita or even with flat bread and you have a healthy home-made lunch or dinner.

Red Lentil Soup

- 1 cup red lentils
- 3 cups water
- 1 small onion, finely chopped
- 1 tablespoon olive oil or vegetable oil
- ½ tsp salt
- 2 to 4 garlic cloves, finely chopped
- 1 bay leaf
- ½ tsp Black Pepper
- Juice of ½ lemon

Directions

Cook lentils with garlic, half chopped onion, salt and pepper for 30 minutes or until the lentils are very soft. Make it smooth using a wooden spoon. Add bay leaves and lemon juice and let the lentil simmer for another 10 minutes. Discard bay leave.

Sauté the leftover onion in oil in a medium heavy saucepan over medium heat, stir occasionally until crispy brown. Add a few cumin seeds to oil.

Pour the mixture over lentil soup. It is ready to be served. You may do it without it if you want to avoid oil but it will not taste so good.

If you want to make it thicker let it stay on high flame for 5 minutes. Keep checking it when it gets thicker turn off the stove. You may serve lentils on rice, with slices of bread, pita or flat bread.

Black Lentil Soup

- 1 cup black lentils (soaked for 2 hours)
- 1 small onion cut finely into small pieces
- 2 garlic cloves crushed finely
- 1 bay leaf
- 1 stalk of celery finely slices
- ¼ red bell pepper cut into small pieces
- ½ spoon of sea salt (make it more or less according to your taste)
- 2 tablespoon of olive oil
- 1 teaspoon of lemon juice
- A few mint leaves finely chopped
- 3 cups of water

Directions

Drain out the water. Put soaked lentil in a big pot and add 3 cups of water. Let it come to boil on high heat then let it simmer on low heat. After 20 minutes add celery, red pepper, bay leaf, garlic, sea salt and half chopped onion. Stir well and let it simmer on medium heat for another 20 minutes or till lentils are very tender and soft. Add the lemon juice and mint leaves. Sauté the leftover onion in oil in a medium heavy saucepan over medium heat, stirring occasionally until onion is crispy brown. Add a few cumin seeds to oil.

Pour the mixture over lentil soup. Eat it as soup, if thicker eat it with rice, flat bread, pita, or just with sliced bread.

Creamy Corn Soup #1

- 2 cans cream-style corn
- 2 eggs, beaten
- 2 tablespoons cornstarch
- 6 cups of water
- 1 cup frozen corn kernel
- salt and black pepper

Directions

In a saucepan combine the creamed corn and water; bring to a boil over medium-high heat. In a cup whisk the cornstarch and water; add to the simmering corn soup and continue to cook for about 1 minute or until thickened.

Add in the frozen corn kernel that should be heated before adding to the soup. Gradually add the beaten eggs while stirring the soup constantly. Season it with salt and pepper. Serve and enjoy!

Creamy Corn Soup #2

- 21 oz vegetable broth
- 8 oz cream style corn 2 tsp olive oil
- I cup frozen corn kernels
- 1 tsp white pepper
- 3 tbsp cornstarch
- 6 cup water
- 3 beaten eggs
- 3 scallion thinly sliced
- ½ cup frozen peas

Directions

Stir together the broth, cream-style corn, olive oil, corn kernels, peas and white pepper in a large saucepan. Bring to a boil over high heat. Dissolve cornstarch into the water and stir into boiling soup. Boil for 30 seconds until soup thickens, stir soup rapidly in one direction, slowly pour in the beaten egg gently stirring it. Stir in the green onions and serve.

Vegetable Soup

- ¼ cup chopped leek
- 1 celery sticks diced
- 1 large carrot cut into small cubes
- 1 large potato cut into small cube
- 1 medium onion diced
- ¼ cup spinach finely chopped
- ½ green bell pepper cubed
- ½ red bell pepper cubed
- 1 tomato, seeded and cut into small cubes
- 1 quart of vegetable (chicken broth)
- 1 tablespoon olive oil
- ¼ teaspoon sage chopped finely
- ¼ cup of cilantro chopped finely
- 4 oz chicken breast pieces (optional)
- ½ teaspoon sea salt
- black pepper to taste

Directions

In a large heavy pot add oil, when heated add onions and leek for I minute then add all the vegetables. Stir a few times then add the broth. Let it simmer for 20 minutes. Add sage and cilantro. Soup is ready to be served with bread slices. It's a full meal. Good in winter.

If you want to add the chicken pieces either grill them or boil in very little water that is absorbed when chicken is done. Add the chicken pieces or you may even shred them before you add them to soup. Serves 4

Beans Soup

There is a large variety of beans; kidney, broad, black eye, chickpeas, lentils, azuki, pinto etc to name the few. And there are varieties of ways to cook them. They are also very low in saturated fat, cholesterol, and sodium. They are good source of vitamins and minerals and also a good source of dietary fiber and folate. Beans are hearty and they make you feel full.

- 1 pre-packed mixed beans soup packet
- ½ medium onion chopped
- 1 bay leaf

- ¼ spoon ground cumin
- ¼ spoon paprika powder
- ¼ spoon garlic paste
- ½ spoon ginger past
- 1 spoon olive oil
- 6 cups water
- Salt to taste, (if anyone in the house is diabetic do not use salt)
- Cilantro leaves to add to soup when served
- For better taste you may add one beef or chicken bouillon cube to the boiling water

Directions

Soak beans overnight. Put a large heavy pan on the stove. Add water to the pot. And keep it on high flame. When water is boiling rinse beans and add them to the pot along with all the ingredients. When again comes to boil reduce heat to low and let the soup simmer for one and half hour or till all the beans are soft and tender. Serve in bowls and add a few cilantro leaves on top.

2. Vegetarian Dishes

Potatoes with Cumin Seeds

- 6 Medium size Potatoes
- 1 tablespoon oil
- ¼ spoon cumin seeds
- 1/8 spoon of crushed red pepper
- ¼ spoon of sea salt (make it more or less according to taste or need)
- Lemon
- Cilantro leaves

Directions

Peel the potatoes and thinly slice them. Use a large and deep frying pan on medium heat. Pour oil in it, when heated add cumin seeds, when they are brown add sliced potatoes, salt and red pepper. Sir well and cover the frying pan with lid. Lower the heat. No need to add any water. Potatoes will be done in 10 minutes. Stir once or twice not to let them stick to frying pan. Squeeze a little lemon on it and garnish with chopped cilantro leaves. Serve as a side dish.

Hummus

- 1 can chickpeas
- 1/3 cup tahini (sesame seeds paste)
- 3 tablespoon olive oil
- 2 tablespoon lemon juice
- 2 clove garlic
- Mint leaves

Directions

Rinse and drain the chickpeas. Combine chickpeas, tahini, lemon juice, 1 clove of garlic and half olive oil in the food processor and blitz it until smooth. Save other clove of garlic for later use. If it is too thick add 1 tablespoon of water to get the right consistency. Serve hummus in a plate. In the center add crushed garlic, pour saved olive oil on it and garnish it with mint leaves.

Rice and Veggie Pilaf

- ½ cup finely chopped onion (1 small)
- 2 tablespoons extra-virgin olive oil
- 1 cup basmati rice
- 2 cup water
- 1/3 cup slivered almonds, toasted
- ½ teaspoon salt
- 3/4 cup frozen mixed vegetables
- ½ spoon garlic paste
- ½ spoon ginger paste
- 1 hot green pepper finely chopped
- Cilantro finely chopped

Directions

Fry onion in oil in a 2-quart heavy saucepan over moderate heat, stirring occasionally, until golden brown, 5 to 7 minutes. Add garlic and ginger paste and vegetables to saucepan and stir a few times (1 minute).

Add rice, salt and 2 cup water and let it come to boil. Lower the heat and let it simmer for 20 minutes, or until rice is soft. Fluff with a fork, and stir in almonds. Serve warm or at room temperature in a platter. Garnish with cilantro and chopped green pepper. Serves 2.

Curried Chickpeas

This simplified version of an Indian favorite is a delightful way to showcase tasty chickpeas. You can also use commercial Chana Masala ingredients, easily available from Indo-Pakistani stores and super markets.

- 2 tablespoon olive oil
- 1 large onion, chopped
- ½ spoon garlic paste
- 2 teaspoons ginger paste
- ½ cup of tomato puree
- 2 cans (16-ounce) of chickpeas, drained and rinsed
- ½ teaspoon turmeric
- ½ teaspoon ground cumin
- ¼ red pepper powder
- ¼ cup minced fresh cilantro, more or less to taste
- Salt to taste
- ¼ teaspoon of baking soda

Directions

Heat the oil in a wide skillet. Add the onion and sauté until translucent. Add garlic and ginger and continue to sauté until the onion is golden.

Add the chickpeas, seasonings, tomatoes, lemon juice, salt and about 1/2 cup water. Add baking soda. Bring to a boil, then on low heat let it simmer, for 20 minutes, stirring frequently. It should be moist but not soupy.

Season with cilantro and chopped green peppers (if like it hot). Serve in shallow bowls. Curried chickpeas may be served with rice or nan (flat bread). Serve: 4 to 6.

Steamed Broccoli

Take one pound broccoli head. Cut it to separate florets. Put 2 tablespoon water in a deep frying pan to boil. Add broccoli florets. Cover the pan. Steam it for 5 minutes. Sprinkle pepper to taste. Add 2 dashes of soy sauce. Serve hot. Serve it as a side dish.

Omelet

Spinach is a common ingredient in a number of egg dishes. Spinach omelet has a distinctive flavor and taste. To make this omelet you'll need:

- ¼ cup finely chopped spinach
- 2 eggs
- 1 small very finely chopped onion
- 1 scallion finely chopped
- Salt
- Pepper
- ¼ cup finely chopped cilantro
- ¼ green bell pepper finely cubed
- 1 pinch of nutmeg

Directions

Add all the ingredients to the bowl with whisked eggs and mix well. Use a 9 inch frying pan. Put 2 tablespoon of olive oil in the frying pan. When the oil is hot pour the whisked eggs in the frying pan and keep it on medium heat. Spread it evenly with spatula or spoon. Cover it for 2 minutes. Omelet is done in steam. If the cover sweats too much take it off and let the omelet be done without covering it. If you need to turn it over you may do so for ½ minute.

More Suggestions

- You may replace spinach with mushrooms, scallion, baby spinach leaves, pitted and halved olives, Cheese etc or any other leafy vegetable. Onions are a basic ingredient in many Asian dishes especially the vegetables. They enhance the nutritional value and the taste of vegetables. Most of the dishes begin with chopped and sautéed onions.

Vegetarian Chilli

- To make vegetarian chilli, use a can of rajma (kidney beans), 6 oz. of chunky tomato sauce, and 2 tablespoons of olive oil, heat together 1 medium chopped sautéed onion, and season to taste with chili powder, cilantro or basil leaves. Add pearl onions raw or grilled to it.

- To make a salsa dip chop 1 red onion, 2 medium tomatoes, 2 avocados and 1hot red pepper and blend them coarsely in the blender. Add a little bit of salt and ¼ spoon of sugar.

Rajma curry (kidney Beans)

- 1 canned Rajma/Red Kidney Beans
- 1 Bay Leaf
- 1 inch Cinnamon piece
- 1 Green Cardamom
- 3 Cloves
- 2 large Onions
- 2 large Tomatoes
- 2 Green Chilli
- 2 tbsp Oil
- ½ tsp Cumin Seeds
- 1/2 tbsp Ginger Paste ½ garlic paste 1 tsp Red Chilli Powder 1/4 tsp Turmeric Powder
- 1/2 tsp Coriander Seeds Powder
- ½ tsp turmarind(imli) paste
- ¼ cup Fanugreek leaves (dried)
- 1 tsp Roasted Cumin Powder
- Salt to Taste
- 2 tbsp Chopped cilantro Leaves—
- A pinch of Asafoetida/ Heeng (it's a digestive substance)
- 1 cup water.

Directions

1. Drain and rinse canned rajma.
2. In a pan heat oil. Add onion and saute until onions become golden brown. Add cumin seeds, cloves, cardamom.
3. Add chili powder, ginger and garlic paste, turmeric, coriander powder and mix well, Add a pinch of of Asafoetida/ Heeng. Stir for a minute. Add water.
4. Now add tomatoes and stir, cover and cook until tomato gets mashed, stir in intervals.
5. Add salt, crushed leaves of fenugreek and turmarind paste, cumin powder, and stir to mix well.

6.   Simmer on low heat for another 5 minutes or until gravy becomes thick.
7.   Garnish with coriander leaves and take the pot off the stove.

Serve warm on a plate of rice. You may serve it with roti, nan (different kinds of flat breads, or fried flat bread (paratha) or even with rolls.
Serve: 3-4

3.   Salads

Chickpea Salad

- 1 cup of chick peas drained and rinsed
- 1 small onion very finely chopped
- 1 medium size potato boiled and cut into small pieces
- ¼ green or red bell pepper cut into small pieces
- ¼ lime or lemon
- Few cilantro leaves chopped finely
- Salt and pepper to taste

Directions

Mix all the ingredients in a bowl and squeeze the lime or lemon on it. It may be served as a side dish or eaten as snack with tea. Serve 2 or 3

Fruity salad

- 1 apple
- 1 pear
- 1 kiwi (if available) Replace kiwi with mango, apricot or an orange
- ½ cup of chick peas drained and rinsed
- 6 baby carrots sliced
- ½ cucumber cut into small pieces
- ½ romaine lettuce sliced or broken into small pieces
- ½ lemon
- 1 table spoon of olive oil
- Sprinkle of salt and black pepper to taste

Directions

Peel and cut apple, pear and kiwi in to small pieces. Slice carrots. Mix fruits, chickpeas, cucumber (sliced) and lettuce (leaves broken into small pieces) in a small bowl. Squeeze the lemon on salad. Add olive oil, salt and black pepper to your taste. (No salt if diabetic or have high blood pressure)

Veggie Salad

- 5 oz. baby spinach leaves
- 1 broccoli
- 8 baby carrots
- 1 apple
- 1 cucumber
- ¼ lemon
- 1 spoon olive oil
- 1 tablespoon of sunflower seeds
- 1 spoon flex seeds
- Salt
- Pepper

Cut apple and cucumber into small pieces. Slice baby carrots. Cut broccoli florets. Mix them in a bowl. Add olive oil. Squeeze the lemon on them. Sprinkle it with some sunflower and flex seeds. Add salt and pepper to taste.

Avocado Salad

- 1 can chickpeas, rinsed and drained
- 1 avocado, cut into small pieces
- ¼ cup cheese, crumbled
- 1 medium onion, thinly sliced
- ¼ cup freshly squeezed lemon juice
- ¼ teaspoon chili powder (if you prefer)
- 1 tablespoon olive oil
- 1 red or green bell pepper, thinly sliced
- ¼ cup cilantro chopped
- ½ teaspoon black pepper or according to taste
- ½ teaspoon salt or according to taste.(no salt for high blood pressure patients)

In a bowl combine chickpeas, avocado, cheese, half of the cilantro, and lemon juice and chili powder. Toss well. Garnish vegetables with rest of the cilantro.

Walnut or Pecan Salad

- 2 cups chopped Romaine lettuce
- 5 celery stalks, chopped
- 1 large pear, cored and cubed
- 2 tablespoons chopped fresh chives
- 1 cup seedless green grapes, halved
- 1 cup cherry tomatoes
- 5 tablespoons nonfat plain Greek yogurt
- 3 tablespoons freshly squeezed lemon juice
- 1 teaspoon mustard
- ¼ teaspoon salt
- ¼ teaspoon black pepper
- 1 cup lightly toasted walnuts or pecan halves. (you may break them into smaller pieces)

Directions

In a large bowl, whisk together yogurt, lemon juice, mustard, salt, pepper and chives. Add pear, lettuce, celery, grapes, cherry tomatoes and walnuts or pecans to bowl and toss to coat. Serve 4.

Pomegranate Salad

- 1 cup pomegranate seeds
- 1 pear
- 1 apple
- 5 oz baby spinach
- ½ romaine lettuce
- ½ chickpeas drained and rinsed
- 1 tbsp lime juice
- ¼ cup sliced almonds or pecans
- 10 big leaves fresh mint thinly sliced

Core and cut in cube apples and pears. Cut lettuce finely. Combine fruits in a salad bowl. Add chickpeas and spinach leaves. Toss well. Drizzle with lime juice and toss again. Sprinkle with sliced almonds or pecans and fresh mint leaves before serving. Top it with pomegranate seeds. Serve 4.

Salad with Shrimps

- 20 shrimps small or medium size pre-cooked that have been peeled, deveined and tails removed
- 2 tablespoons extra-virgin olive oil
- 2 tablespoons apple cider vinegar
- 1 tablespoon chopped fresh cilantro
- 1 5-ounce bag baby spinach
- 1 cup grape tomatoes, halved
- 1 small red onion, thinly sliced
- 8 pitted olives, halved or quartered

Directions

In a large bowl, whisk together oil, vinegar, cilantro. Add spinach, tomatoes, onion and olives and toss to coat. Divide among four plates and top each with 5 shrimp. Serves 4.

Scallion Salad with Red and Green Peppers

- 2 scallion, chopped
- ½ red pepper cut into very small pieces
- ½ green bell pepper cut into small pieces
- 4 large tomatoes, cored and cut into chunks
- 1 apple, peeled and cut into small pieces
- 3 tablespoons freshly squeezed lemon juice
- 2 tablespoons extra-virgin olive oil
- ½ teaspoon salt (less for HBP patients)
- ½ teaspoon black pepper
- 1 cup flat-leaf parsley leaves or cilantro leaves

Directions

In a large bowl, whisk together oil, lemon juice, salt and pepper. Add tomatoes, peppers, parsley or cilantro, scallion and apple to bowl and toss to coat. Sprinkle salt and pepper and serve salad on the side with any meat dish.

4. Meat Dishes

People eat meat for its best source of protein. It is also tasty and variety of it is easily available. Meat dishes are delicious, filling and to some people most desirable source of foods. The amount of protein we get from different kind of meat:

- 100g. of Beef has 36g of protein
- 100 grams of cooked chicken meat has about 33 grams of protein
- 1 large egg has 6 grams of protein

Most fish fillets or steaks have about 22 grams of protein for 100 grams of cooked fish,

- Tuna in a 6 oz can has about 40 grams of protein

On the other hand many vegetarian dishes are also very delicious and a very good source of vegetarian protein. We never think of vegetables and greens to be associated with protein but surprisingly many of them have good amount of protein.

A 100-calorie portion of sirloin steak has 5.4 grams of protein, and a 100-calorie portion of broccoli has 11.2 grams of protein.

Cauliflower has 32% protein
Mushrooms have 56% protein
Green pepper has 22% protein
Broccoli 33%
Kale has 26%
Zucchini 30%

Chicken with Basmati Rice and Peas

- 1/3 cup low-fat plain yogurt
- 2 teaspoons freshly squeezed lime juice
- 2 teaspoons garam masala*
- 2 teaspoons olive oil
- ½ teaspoon turmeric
- ¾ teaspoon salt
- ¼ teaspoon garlic powder
- 1/8 teaspoon cayenne pepper

- 4 to 6 ounces boneless, skinless chicken breasts
- Nonstick cooking spray
- 2 cups basmati rice
- 1 cup frozen peas
- 2 tablespoons chopped fresh cilantro (optional)

Directions

1. Preheat the broiler. Combine yogurt, lime juice, garam masala, oil, turmeric, salt, garlic powder and cayenne pepper in a large bowl. Make three diagonal slashes across the top of each chicken breast. Coat chicken pieces with yogurt mixture. Arrange chicken top side down on a foil-lined broiler pan; spray with cooking spray. Broil 4 minutes, flip, spray tops and broil 4 to 6 minutes more or until just cooked through.

2. While chicken is broiling, cook rice with 4 cups of water, ¼ teaspoon salt, 1 tablespoon oil and a bay leaf bring it to boil then let it simmer on low heat for approximately 10 minutes. Mirowave frozen peas according to package directions. Gently combine rice and peas in a big platter. Top with chicken. Garnish with cilantro.

* Garam masala is a mixture of many ground spices: cloves, black pepper, cinnamon, black cardamom, and black cumin seeds. It's like Asian style "All spice" but very aromatic. It is available in all Indian stores. Serve: 4.

Steak with Green Beans and Potatoes

- 1 pound baby potatoes
- 12 ounces green beans (frozen)
- 1 pound skirt steak, (use meat tenderizer for quick cooking)
- ¼ teaspoon salt
- ¼ teaspoon black pepper
- 1 tablespoon red apple vinegar
- 1 teaspoon ginger paste
- 1 teaspoon of garlic paste
- 1 teaspoon sugar
- 4 tablespoons vegetable oil
- ½ teaspoon sesame seeds
- 1/3 cup thinly sliced cilantro

Directions

1. Microwave potatoes on high 5 to 6 minutes or until potatoes are fork-tender. Microwave green beans according to package directions.
2. Heat a pan over medium-high heat. Coat with oil; smear garlic paste on steak and season it with salt and pepper and cook about 8 to 10 minutes turning to the other side after 4 or 5 minutes or until it is done well. Transfer to a cutting board to rest.
3. While steak is cooking, put vinegar, ginger, sugar and rest of the oil in a small bowl to make dressing. Whisk it smooth.
4. Cut potatoes in quarters, and then cut steak into slices. Serve in a big platter with potatoes and beans on the side. Drizzle with dressing. Sprinkle cilantro over steak and sesame seeds over potatoes. Serve: 4

Chicken Meatballs on Pasta or rice

- 1 pound ground chicken
- 2 small onions, finely chopped
- 1/2 teaspoon sea salt
- 2 teaspoons vegetable oil
- 1 tablespoon ginger paste
- 1 teaspoon ground coriander
- ¼ teaspoon ground turmeric
- **½ spoon red pepper powder**
- 4 oz tomato sauce
- 2 bay leaves
- Cilantro leaves
- 2 slices of whole-wheat bread

Directions

1. In a medium bowl, combine chicken, scallions, 1/4th ginger and 1/2 teaspoon salt. Mix well and form chicken into 12 meatballs.
2. In a large skillet, heat oil over medium-high heat. Add 1 cup of water or broth, tomato sauce, ginger, coriander and turmeric stirring constantly, add red pepper powder, bay leaves and remaining salt; bring to a boil, then reduce heat to low. Add meatballs and simmer until meat balls are tender and

cooked thoroughly, about10 to 15 minutes. Top with cilantro leaves if desired.

3. Serve with any kind of pasta, pita bread, noodles or rice. You may even serve meatballs with mashed potatoes. Serves 4.

Chicken Biryani

It's a famous Indian sub-continental dish. It's a meal in itself. It can be served with yogurt raita, salad, and with any other chicken or meat dish.

- 2 lb chicken cut into small pieces
- ½ cup oil
- 1/2 cup whipped yogurt
- 1 large onion
- 1 teaspoon ginger paste
- 1 teaspoon garlic paste
- 4 cloves
- 4 whole black pepper
- 3 cardamom
- 2 inch piece of cinnamon
- ¼ spoon cumin powder
- ½ spoon coriander powder
- ½ red chili powder
- Saffron or orange food color
- I bay leaf
- 2 cups basmati rice
- A few cilantro and mint leaves to garnish

Directions

Heat oil and fry sliced onions. When crispy brown take out half of them and keep them aside. Add ginger and garlic paste, cloves, black pepper and salt and chicken pieces to the pot. Stir a few times and let the chicken pieces become brownish. Add yogurt stir occasionally till yogurt water is absorbed. Add cumin and coriander powder, red chili powder and stir to mix all spices well. Add very little water if needed to get the chicken tender. Add cinnamon and 4 cardamoms. Let it simmer till the chicken is tender and most of the water is evaporated.

Soak the rice ½ hour earlier. Now in other pot boil 3 and 3/4 cups of water, add bay leaf and 2 cardamoms. Add rice to boiling water.

When boiling turn the heat to low and the rice will be done in about 15-20 minutes. If rice is not tender enough sprinkle about 2 tablespoon of milk, cover the pot and let it stay on very low heat for 5 minutes. Turn off the stove. Layer the rice and curried meat in layers.

To give color to some of the rice mix orange food color in a bowl with water or milk and drop it on different places so it will penetrate all the way down to the bottom of the pot. Take biryani out in a big platter. Garnish with cilantro and/or mint leaves. Spread out the saved fried onion on the biryani.

Biryani can be served with Yogurt Raita, plain yogurt or with any meat dish with gravy.

How to Make Yogurt Raita

- 1 cup yogurt whisked
- ¼ spoon cumin powder
- ¼ spoon salt
- ¼ green bell pepper and cilantro leaves

Blend all the ingredients in the blender coarsely and mix them in the yogurt. If you do not like yogurt raita too thick add 2 or 3 spoons of milk or water in it.

Fried Fish

- 2 fillets of Basa fish
- ½ spoon garlic paste
- Salt
- Pepper
- Lemon juice
- Whole wheat flour
- Red apple cider vinegar
- Oil

Directions

Soak fresh Basa fillet in 2 spoons of vinegar and sprinkle some salt on it. In 2 minutes rinse it and dry it with paper towels. Cut the fillet in length and cut the strip in 2. That gives you 8 pieces. Mix lemon juice, garlic paste, salt and pepper and coat the fish pieces with this mixture on both sides. Use a deep frying pan to fry fish pieces. Put the frying pan on medium-high flame. When the oil is heated take each piece of fish coat it with flour and fry it. Place them on paper towel to absorb access oil.

Different Version of Fried Fish

Prepare fish as above. But keep the fillets without cutting into pieces. You may bake the 2 big fillets of Basa fish or use shallow frying pan with one spoon of olive oil. It will be done in 5 minutes on stove top.

You can also try tilapia fillets the same way. It will take a little longer time to get done.

Ground Chicken (qeema)

- 1 lb ground chicken, (beef, goat or any other meat you prefer)
- 4 tablespoon vegetable oil
- 2 medium size tomatoes
- 3 medium size onions, about ¾ lb
- 8 cloves of garlic
- 2 inch piece of fresh ginger
- 1 spoon garam masala (Allspice)
- Salt
- Red chili powder
- Green pepper
- Cilantro

Directions

Heat oil and fry onions till golden brown. Add, ginger, garlic and 2 onions. Add ground meat, and continue to stir till it changes color, or for 2 minutes. Add salt, red chili pepper and tomatoes. When tomatoes are tender and their water is absorbed stir a few times to get all ingredients mixed well.

Chicken ground meat may be done without adding any water. Add ½ cup of water if it is beef. Cover the pan and let it simmer for 15 minutes. If needed just add 1 tablespoon of water more.

Take out in a serving dish, garnish with green pepper and cilantro. Cut third onion into rings and spread it on ground meat.

Variations

You may add potatoes, beans, peas, spinach, cauliflower or any other vegetable of your choice. You may also cook these vegetables separately and serve as side dish.

Ground meat can also be served with rice, pasta or pita bread.

5. How to Reduce Weight Naturally

Obesity is like a disease and is risky for your health. Before your weight goes out of control start thinking of ways how you can control it. Actually it is very difficult to lose weight if you have put on too much already. To stay healthy and risk-free of heart attack and other diseases you have to watch it when you start gaining weight. There are many ways of reducing and controlling it. First thing is to modify your diet.

- Eat fruits and green vegetables as they are low in calories. If you are overweight you should use fruits and vegetables more frequently in your diet.
- Avoid taking too much salt. Salt may be a factor for increasing the body weight.
- Cut down milk products like cheese, butter because these are rich in fat.
- Avoid eating meat and any non-vegetarian foods.
- Use spices like ginger, cinnamon, black pepper etc. for losing weight. They can be used in a number of ways.
- Vegetables like bitter gourd (Karela), are useful for losing weight.
- Taking honey is an excellent home remedy for obesity. It mobilizes the extra deposited fat in the body and puts it into circulation, which is utilized as energy for normal functions. Take one spoon of honey in hot water early in the morning.
- Drinking lemon water in the morning is very good for reducing weight.
- Cabbage is considered to be an effective remedy for losing weight. This vegetable inhibits the conversion of sugar and other carbohydrates into fat. Hence, it is of great value in weight reduction. It can be taken raw or cooked.
- Exercise is an important part of weight reduction plan. It helps to use up calories stored in body as fat. In addition, it also

relieves tension and tones up the muscles of the body. Walking is the best exercise to begin with and may be followed by running, swimming, rowing.

- Lime juice is excellent for weight reduction. Juice of a lime mixed in a glass of warm water and sweetened with honey should be taken every morning on an empty stomach.
- Measure the portions of your food every meal and make sure that the portions are small. For example one portion of rice should not be more than the quantity which can fit in your fist. Smaller meals at a regular interval of 4 to 5 hours will keep your metabolism high and prevent your body from converting the food you intake into fat.
- You must also include regular exercise in your daily routine to help enhance weight reduction.

6. Carrot Juice

Carrot juice is the richest source of vitamin A. The body can easily assimilate this type of vitamin A. Carrot juice also has a good supply of vitamins B, C, D, E, G, and K.

Benefits of drinking carrot juice:

- It is a juice you can drink every day. In place of orange juice you may drink a glass of carrot juice. Without mixing any other fruit juices carrot juice is sweet enough to drink and is potent all by itself. The carrot juice molecule is like the blood molecule. Maybe this is one of the main reasons why carrot juice is so beneficial for the body.
- Carrot juice helps in improving and maintaining the bone structure of the teeth.
- It helps nursing mothers enhance milk quality.
- It helps prevent infections of the eyes and throat, as well as tonsils and sinuses and the respiratory organs.
- Vitamin K in carrot juice helps eye sight. It nourishes the optic system.
- Carrot juice nourishes the entire system.
- It helps normalizes chemical balance in the body.
- It also helps control weight.
- It helps with dry skin, dermatitis, and other skin blemishes.

7. Foods that Boost Your Brain and Memory

There are many foods that help boost your memory and brain. In old age when most of the people start losing their short term memory they will be especially helpful. After a long illness it is advisable to make use of these foods to enhance your memory and brain function.

- Apples are power food for mind, body, and emotions.
- Avocados, apples, dark chocolate, green tea, and blueberries are very helpful in boosting memory.
- Blueberries improve learning and motor skills. They bring vitality in the body.
- Watermelon targets brain function and hydrates the body.
  These are in the category of fruits that help brain function and the memory.

- Walnuts are high in omega 3.
- Almonds increase blood flow to the brain.
  These nuts are also very helpful for brain function.

- Brussels sprout has tryptophan which converts to seroten that is good for brain health.
- Broccoli assists in brain functioning. Steamed broccoli is the best way of consuming it.
- Cauliflower assists in cleansing white matter in brain.
- Cabbage is considered a help in lowering risk of brain, lung, and prostate cancer.
- Lettuce helps increase blood flow to the brain.
  These vegetables if are used regularly will enhance memory and increase blood flow to the brain, hence the brain activity.
  Ginger is anti inflammatory. It is of all the herbs and roots the most important herb. It is used in many ailments and regular use of ginger in our foods helps in healing any inflammation in the body and mind.

If you have deficiency of potassium, which you only find out from your blood test report that your doctor orders for you. Then the following foods will help you increase the potassium level in your blood. Almonds, apricots and avocados

- Bok Choy, broccoli, Brussel sprouts, beets, spinach, Swiss chard, and tomatoes are the vegetables that are very rich in potassium.
- Figs and Kiwi and Cantaloupe are the fruits that should be recommended to increase potassium in blood.
- Brazil nuts and coconut also provide potassium.

References

1. Pesmen, Curt, Bottom Line/Health, Uncommon cures for everyday ailments (2010)
2. Michael Castleman, The New healing herbs (2001)
3. Dr. Fife, Bruce, Director of the Coconut Research Center, Article: Coconut "The Tree of Life."
4. Meyer, Clarence, American Folk Medicine, (1973)
5. Bottom Line Publications, The World's Greatest Treasury of health Secrets (2010) *http://www.wikipedia.org*
6. Lynley Kempthorne: organic Facts-Dates *http://www.livestrong.com,*
7. Katherine Zeratsky, R.D., L.D (Mayo Clinic.) *http://www.mayoclinic.com,*
8. University of Maryland Medical Center, Green tea | *http://umm.edu/health/medical/altmed/herb/green-tea#ixzz2jV474NQ0*
9. Lindsey Duncan, ND, CN, Honey's Unknown Benefits, *http://www.doctoroz.com/expert/lindsey-duncan*
10. Robbie Robbins M.D., D.D.S. FAAOHNS Robbins Family Farm